ELDER
A SPIRITUAL ALTERNATIVE TO BEING ELDERLY

Terry Jones D.Min.

Elderhood Institute Books

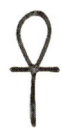

ELDER

Copyright © 2006 by Terry Jones.

All rights reserved.

Elderhood Institute Books
516 SE Morrison St. Suite 1110
Portland, OR 97214
www.elderhood.org

Cover photo: Kevin Connors, www.kconnors.com
Cover and page design: Anita Jones and Joan Pinkert

Printed in the United States of America
First Printing: March, 2006
10 9 8 7 6 5 4 3 2 1

Library of Congress-in-Publication Data

Elder: A Spiritual Alternative to Being Elderly
Terry Jones

   p.   cm.
Includes bibliographical references.
  ISBN 1-59975-671-4
  1. Aged — Attitudes. 2. Old Age — Psychological aspects.
3. Self-actualization (Psychology) in old age
I. Title

HQ1061. J53 2006
  305.31 — dc21

Order this book at www.elderhood.org or call Elderhood Institute at 800-854-9968 E. 302

ISBN 10: 1-59975-671-4
ISBN 13: 978-1-59975-671-4

*Elder is dedicated to the magnificent seven
and also to their magnificent seven,
Josh, Val, Alyssa, Trinity, Chloe,
Olivia and Noah.*

Contents

Preface i
Introduction v

CHAPTER ONE
Elders As Spiritual Models 1
    One Elder 2
    Spiritual Journey 3
    The Four Paths 5
    Blessing by Elders 8
    Elderhood 13
    My Search 16
    Elders and the Aged Lose Credibility 18
    Elders as Victims of Progress 27
    Mentoring 30
    Retirement 35
    Wisdomkeeping 37
    Earthkeeping 39

CHAPTER TWO
The Elder in History 43
    Biblical Elders 45
    The Crone 48

Magic and the Elder 49
  Oral Tradition 50
  Far Eastern Elderhood..53
  Indigenous History 56
  Hermits 60
  Decline of the Elder 61
  Wisdom in History...67
  The Renaissance 70
  Modern History 73

CHAPTER THREE
Elder Roles And Archetypes 79
  20th Century 81
  21st Century 83
  Roles As Archetypes 84
  Sovereign, Lover, Warrior, Magician 87
  Sovereign..91
  Lover 93
  Warrior..95
  Magician 97
  The Masculine and the Feminine 100

CHAPTER FOUR
Elder as Revived Child..103
  Child/Elder Archetypes 106
  Recalling Childhood 108
  Adultism 110
  Elders and Children Are Look-alikes 112
  Heidi and the Alm Uncle 114
  Play and Creativity 119

CHAPTER FIVE
Eldering as Maturity 123
  The Three Challenges 127
  A Revolution of Spirit 131
  Immaturity at Work...134

CHAPTER SIX
Becoming an Elder 141
- Elderhood as a Stage of Personal Growth 142
- The Initiation of An Elder 151
- Initiation Process 155
- Growing Into Elderhood 164
- Accessibility 166
- Celebration 166
- Forgiveness 168
- Confronting Our Mortality 169
- Developing Confidence in Your Wisdom 171
- Loosening Our Grip 173
- Balancing Our Psychic Energies 175
- Elder Council 178

CHAPTER SEVEN
Action Elderhood 181
- Giving Attention, Being Accessible 182
- Facilitating Community 183
- Advocating for Family 185
- Passing It On 187
- Modeling Good Health 188
- Protector Roles for Elders 189
- Stewardship 190
- A Soul Nourishing Pace 191
- Protecting Through Blessing 193
- Heeding Those Without Hope 195
- Increasing Levels of Elder Action 196
- Elders As Teachers 198
- Passing On A Legacy 198
- Reaching Out to Younger People 199

References 203

Index 213

Preface

*O*nce *elders were linked to the magic of the cosmos. The mature ones were* the source of blessings and taught young people about the mystery of our oneness with the universe. They fostered an oral tradition and offered wisdom to younger folks. What happened?

With the advent of the Industrial Era, people began leaving farms and villages to work in factories. Soon elders became simply "the elderly"; all too often portraying a negative model of aging that leads only to seclusion, pain and a fear of or longing for the end of life. The elderly grew more distant from the young and became characterized by words such as "disengagement" and "retirement". Our pattern for the past three hundred years has been to reach the zenith of our influence in midlife, then give way to an inevitable decline as we grow older. For too long, we have confused "old" with unhappy, frustrated, impotent, and weak. The second half of life, however, need not be a time of depletion emotionally, intellectually and spiritually.

In *Elder* you will discover a generative model for moving from "adulthood" to "elderhood". Older people today are fully capable of rediscovering their spiritual radiance and maintaining their social responsibilities as wisdomkeepers, earthkeepers, mentors and celebrants, sources of blessing.

When I first learned about elderhood and its opportunities and responsibilities, I wanted to meet some of those people who had embraced this nurturing role. They are hard to find so I went in search of them.

I listed what I felt were qualities of an elder, wrote them down and carried them in my wallet. My card said an elder is someone who:

- *Is seasoned, and a source of life-giving energy*
- *Knows their limitations and is skillful*
- *Has an unconquerable spirit*
- *Is knowledgeable, aware and filled with insight*
- *Is intuitive, passionate, spiritual and sensuous*

I went from person to person asking if anyone knew men who fit that description.

In that my research at that earlier time was primarily about men I wrote a book entitled *The Elder Within: The Source of Mature Masculinity*. I identified many men and women deserving of the title of elder, although few of them cared to claim their elderhood. An elder is not, I discovered, an example of a perfect person, or even a completely balanced one. I have gained increasing hope, therefore, that most people could, over time, become more elder like. I believe an elder is any older person who is committed to sharing her or his wisdom and remaining accessible to those who might be served and she or he is willing to let go of their biases about aging and confront their mortality. Anyone willing to forgive those who harmed them and release the wasted energy used for holding grudges can embrace elderhood, that spiritual stage of development that comes after adulthood. Elders seek out the young to be an advocate for them and make their life journey more meaningful.

My search for elders developed into a passion. I have discovered that older people throughout early history often evolved into a role called elder in the second half of life. The role of the elder differs from what we call today, the elderly. Many of today's elderly feel angry and hurt and live with fear. Some seem to be waiting for their life to end. Too many of our elderly today actually scare the young and reinforce the bias we grow up with about aging as impotency and/or crankiness. But this was not always so. As far back as recorded history, most communities honored their senior members. The second half of life was for many older people a time not of retirement but of service. Elders were the master craftspeople, the wise aunt, the generative minister, and the teachers who were devoted to their pupil's dreams. They were the *sannyasin* in India, the loving *sheik* in Islam, the devoted grandfather and the Desert Fathers and Mothers of the early Christian church who made themselves accessible to those hungry to develop a spiritual life.

I wrote this book because I am still looking at just how grown-up I am at age 65. I became a seminar leader for the Spiritual Eldering Institute in 1998, one of the only national organizations that address the concept of elder directly. In 2000 I also became certified as a spiritual director because, at least for me, the training was elder training. It was focused on qualities such as discernment and advocating the spiritual expression of others. In 2001 I called together a body of men and women to form what we call, the Elder Council. In this sacred circle, I receive the support of others ages 50 to 90 who are trying to celebrate their long life by giving back to the community. This book, like *The Elder Within*, is about my considerations concerning elderhood and what I have learned about it that can be utilized by anyone wanting to become creative and generative after 65. Now as I embrace the experience of being a grandfather, a retired mental health consultant, writer and gardener, I have an uncontrollable need to deepen spiritually, to understand how to harvest my life experience, and increasingly be accessible to my family and my community.

I wrote *Elder*, because I am discovering something new in my life. Throughout my life I have written down thoughts on new life challenges. When, 33 years ago, my wife and I were birthing our children, I became enamored with the role of expectant fathers. I self-published a handbook for expectant fathers. When I did my research in graduate school for my master's thesis in history, I came across a little known Japanese-American, Kanaye Nagasawa, and eventually co-authored a book about his life. Paul Kadota and I published the book in Japan. When, in 1979, I opened one of the first firms devoted to providing counseling services to business and industry in Northwestern USA, I wrote and published a handbook for employers entitled, *Employee Assistance Programs in Industry.*

As I have delved into the concept of what it means to be an elder, I have been both fed and left hungry. I am fed by the hopeful potential of elderhood as a way of being in the second half of life. I am hungry for the acceptance of the idea of elderhood. I believe I am living in a time when a new paradigm of aging can emerge. To many people it is too tiring to consider a celebration of one's wisdom and long life experience. The only paradigm we have been offered is called "retirement". To the young in this culture, the idea of utilizing older people as mentors is unfamiliar. Those inclined to "eldering" will have to prove themselves to the young. If we take our retirement money and leave town to see the world but never come back to the community, a long life could be wasted. Eldering could be the answer to the question, "What do we do with the extraordinary long time between ages 60 and 100?"

The first part of the answer to this question is for me a spiritual one. My spirituality has gained considerably more focus ever since I left active employment in 1995. I have come to know myself better physically and emotionally as well but accessing my center, that place that connects me to other people and to the universe is what excites me. In 2005 I graduated from the Doctor of Ministry program at the University of Creation Spirituality (UCS) in Oakland, California. What I have accomplished most of all in this program has been to form my spiritual beliefs into more language that I can share with those I love. Matthew Fox, an Episcopal priest and founder of UCS, largely taught the "language" of Creation Spirituality. The reader will come across this language throughout *Elder*.

Venturing into the world of elderhood is a paradox. While it is new for many of us, eldering is based on an ancient tradition from many cultures. In North America our founding mothers and fathers often understood the role of the loving and balanced older people called elders. But, shortly after fighting for independence, laying the groundwork for the North American version of the Industrial Era and creating a land of the free and a home for the brave, the value of elder energy diminished with the increasing pace of progress. This book sets out to modernize the concept of elderhood for the 21st Century. Imagine, as you read this book, that you will one day be ready to assume the role of elder.

Introduction

As I approached the age of 50, my interests began to shift away from a quest for position, away from molding my children, away from competition and away from "doing" for its own sake. The experience of midlife caused me to consider my mortality. My maternal grandfather lived to age 55. My paternal, to age 74. My father, who is 85 at this writing, will probably live to see 90. Would I live to be 100? I asked myself "What was my role going to be in this long second half of life?"

I had spent the better part of half a century striving for success, ensuring that I provided for my family, being a responsive husband and effective father to my six children. However, I judged that my work required competing with others for position and power. In the course of work, I had ignored my health, gained too much weight, and I had chronic back strain. My risk for heart disease increased with elevated cholesterol and blood pressure. I had not allowed time to build friendships. My lifestyle was constructed on assumptions common to other entrepreneurs. These included the belief that I had to attain my professional and financial success before I got too old. I assumed that my credibility as a vital and contributing citizen would begin to diminish once my hair turned gray. I bought into the American perception of older people as a doddering, powerless lot. There are exceptions. We admired Bob Hope and still consider Sophia Loren sexy. Yet for every Tony Bennett, whose age has only added to his icon status, there are a million senior citizens that will never be celebrities. Society merely considers them old.

At age 50, things began to happen to me that led me to ask myself about my potency, image and value. Was I entering a stage of life where I was to be seen as an "old man"? I was left with a void, an emptiness inside that I needed to fill. I was out of balance—physically, intellectually, emotionally and spiritually. About this time of my life my balance was rocked by three major life events: the marriage of my youngest daughter, the discovery of a new passion and the subsequent impact of my new passion had on my professional life.

When my daughter married, she seemed fulfilled in the way I was when I married her mother 25 years earlier. She accomplished it by making a commitment to her soul mate. I was learning for the first time how hard it was to let go of a child and celebrate at the same time. This was the end of my love affair with my daughter as a twosome. I fell in love with my new son-in-law, too, thus creating a threesome. This was for me, both a new start and an ending—a message about mortality. Shortly after the wedding she graduated from college. The family gathered together at commencement to hear her graduation talk. She ended her talk by announcing who the most influential people in her life were. While she mentioned my name, when she got to her new husband, she described him as "the person who completed her!" When I realized that I couldn't have that position in her life, the grieving that began at her wedding took a deeper dip.

The next "aha" hit me when I realized I was not as energized by my work as I had previously been. I had founded a business and begun building my career about 30 years earlier. At age 50, however, I found myself depending more and more on my staff to maintain the day-to-day management of the company. Almost overnight I had lost passion for the work. We were all caught off guard. To my surprise, what became painfully clear was that I was not as essential to the business's success as I had been. I had hired and built a staff of creative and energetic people who brought youthful vigor and imagination to the operation of the company.

I began a search for a different way of being. When the search began I spent about a year letting go of the passion I had for my profession. This was another ending, a transition that made it possible for me to pursue my search but, nevertheless, a transition that required grieving, a letting go once again. I began writing *The Elder Within* then and forming a dream about people in the second half of life.

My drive for prominence, influence and control began shifting into a quieter, less aggressive energy. I have found that this shift is common to many people after mid-life. I wanted less to lead, to make decisions or to attain more status. My parenting approach had shifted away from "in your face" and more toward advocacy from a greater distance. My children were becoming adults and needed me within reach but no longer needed their mother and me to build the railings and define the boundaries. Performing, executing, transacting, discharging and achieving had been core to my use of energy most of my adult life. In my fifties I had begun to feel a hunger for just being present, quieter and celebrating long life. This all spoke to me about spiritual hunger.

My new passion, the search for a more elder-like expression is the subject of this book. This is a search both in the world and inside me. I imagine Americans as they enter retirement taking on roles such as mentor, conservationist, storytellers and sources of blessing. Most of us, however, don't have models for how to utilize the expanded life span that is available to us in the 21st Century. We lose ourselves in work for most of our adult lives. Like our fathers before us, many of us, both men and women who have had careers, have been emotionally distant from our children. We are less skilled in nurturing our spirit. About the same time the changes I mentioned above were occurring, I got involved in the Men's Movement.

I wanted to understand what being a man meant in the second half of life. I participated in ritualized weekend workshops and ongoing men's groups. I learned that like me, men of all ages shared a hunger for spiritual and emotional growth. Many of us missed the nurturing only a father can bring because our fathers were unskilled in connecting to us emotionally. It was in these men's gatherings that I was reminded about the elder. The older men present for the weekends came to be known as the elders. They tried to fill a vacuum left after two centuries of diminishing credibility for elders. I came across women's groups who embraced the archetype of crone. As you will read later on in this book, the crone is one model for elderhood in older women. The elders of pre-industrial communities had been more available to the young because they were not mobile. People were born in and raised in the same community in which they aged and died.

In the 18th Century families became detached from family and community as they moved from farm to factory. Competing for jobs, men forgot the joy of collaboration. In order to survive they learned how to assert power in the workplace. Then they returned to their homes and allowed their power to darken the nature of fatherhood. In these pre-industrial times, men utilized archetypal warrior power to protect their homes and families. Later, the industrialized male used the same power to compete for position. We assured our economic survival by creating an emotional armor that, because of its rigidity, surprisingly led to a greater personal vulnerability. In time women were to join them.

As I began to look for workshops, schools and retreat experiences that could assist me in a stirring of my spirit, I found mostly women in those places. They are many of the spiritual teachers. Fewer women have compromised their soul in competitive and power oriented work environments but it tempts many of them the way it does men. Many women have birthed children and experienced the mystery of creating life. For the most part, women are conscious of their bodies; more completely express emotion and intellectually are eclectic. I believe they have a greater balance between the fourfold aspects of self: physical, spiritual, psychological and intellectual. There are women who, once overwhelmed by their masculine energy, don't fit my bias, however. There also are men who are extraordinarily influenced by their feminine side and are able to ground themselves spiritually. In large part, however, I find as a man that the fourfold balance of life is harder to attain.

Ancient civilizations celebrated the uniqueness of both genders. They often related the two to the ongoing dance of natural phenomena: earth and sky, land and sea, rain and soil. When we modernized the world with machines, we revised the historical roles of men and women. In this book, I treat the transition in gender roles in the same way that social scientists consider most change with its four stages: shock, resistance, exploration, and adaptation. The Industrial Revolution of the 18th and 19th centuries was the shock stage for the historical expression of healthy masculinity and femininity. In the 20th Century women led us through decades of resistance to the devastation of immature male abuse. Women attacked the "feminine mystique" and the inclination of some men to dispossess women of their rights to equality.

The 21st Century could be an experiment in the exploration and adaptation stages of change to a more generative role for older men and women. The prejudice in this culture about aging, combined with an increasing divorce rate, has separated children from their grandparents. With industrialization came an increasing lack of respect for older mentors who could not teach survival in factories that did not exist when they were learning a trade. Only the young could survive under the demands of the factory. With immigration and the separation of older people from their ancestral homes, men turned increasingly to their peers for support and training.

Boys and girls grew up without the initiation to adulthood that the young received in the older, rural community. Older people used to teach younger ones their skills and offered the magic of presence that came with being in the energy field of a mentor. Busy professional women may have not lost a passion for mentoring the young. The ability to bear a child is compelling and usually leads to advocacy for children. However, both men and women in the West have submitted to a bias against older people that has discouraged us from embracing the role of elder as it was seen expressed in simpler days.

This book is an exploration into the potential of elder like expression, the second half of life adventure in celebrating long life, passing on a legacy and advocacy for the young. You will read here that elder means being a "steward of life", both human life and the life of our planet. An elder seeks to affirm life by embracing the ancient archetype of the elder within. Elders foster consensus rather than conflict and competition. They energize themselves through use of the tools of wisdom: meditation, contemplation, and listening. They accept their mortality and honor their body, which they understand is slowly in depletion. With this knowledge they model taking care of themselves, a particularly uncommon trait for the North American male in particular. Most of all, the person who embraces the role of elder makes themselves available to younger people, to the family and to the community. They have confidence in the fruits of long life experience and want to seed the future by sharing with the young. This book is not about becoming an elder as much as going within oneself to stir elder energy and change one's behavior.

In Chapter One you will read about the power of the elder's blessing, the affirmation that says the elder is making an active commitment to assist us in obtaining our dream. Any person inclined to serve society in the second half of life is embracing a key aspect of elderhood. Because few elder models exist, Western people assume that the second half of life means resting, declining in health and becoming useless. An elder's depletion is only physical, however. They address old age by reaping what has been sown rather than whining about reduced strength. In this chapter, I will review the decline of the elder's credibility over the past few centuries and consider the concept of elder as a victim of progress. You will read about the potential and meaning of mentoring, and how "mentor" is a new role that came out of the Industrial Era as a substitute for elder.

Chapter Two is a review of the history of elders. You will read about ancient elders, like those of Moses' time, primitive elders found in indigenous cultures, and the conversion from generative elderhood to the exploitation of patriarchy. Out of the Christian era came a number of spiritual men and women who modeled some aspects of elderhood. However, they lost the trust of younger people by getting caught up in a hunger for power. Some consideration is given to the wise man and the crone as two older expressions of elder. The Renaissance is reviewed with an eye toward this era's emphasis on youth. Society had less appreciation for elderhood in the 16th Century than at any other time in history. The oppressive gerontocracy of more recent history is considered in Chapter Two as a major cause for emigration to the New World.

In Chapter Three, I speculate about the potential of utilizing archetypes of masculinity and femininity in world history as a base for a redefined expression that works in the 21st Century. It is in this chapter that I introduce the concepts of psychoanalyst Carl Jung. He called his historical masculine and feminine models archetypes. We can find them in written myth and stories, and in psychic energy in the collective unconscious. We consider four archetypes of masculinity: Sovereign, Lover, Warrior and Magician. Each archetype has a positive and a negative energy. Understanding and taking charge of both the positive energy, and what Jung called shadow energy, is the success of the mature person. Another challenge is converting the way we played traditional gender roles historically into a 21st Century application. I will assert that maturity includes integrating both masculine and feminine traits into the expression of self.

In Chapters Four and Five elderhood is considered both as a condition of mature expression and alternatively as an expression of our childlike nature.

In Chapter Six, I offer processes that encourage growth into elderhood. The first embraces elderhood as a stage of human development. "Growing up" gets us there. Next, I offer a design for an initiation into the role of elder that takes no less than six months to complete and takes the initiate through the three stages of most rites of passage: separation, threshold and incorporation. Initiation is the process of introducing some-thing new and demonstrating it to someone else. The third and most complex process discussed in Chapter Six is to do the intellectual, psychological and spiritual work necessary to grow into elderhood. In Chapters Six and Seven, the reader will find information on how to become elder like.

Chapter Seven is called "Action Elderhood", not because the world needs aged activists but because elder expression is known to the world by its works. The elder is a spiritual person who believes that he or she exists for a reason. Their search for the reason is what I call the spiritual journey. This journey takes action elders where they can serve others, empower and bless others. At the same time the person who is more elder like honors the reality that each day brings them closer to death than they were when they were "action youths". Action elderhood moves the heart more than the legs. The elder gleans the energy they need from their contemplative activity. The older they get, the more they become acquainted with their spiritual center. Action elderhood is the route to how mature people can play these roles in the 21st Century.

CHAPTER ONE

Elders As Spiritual Models

*T**he second half of a person's life can be an adventure in elderhood: a life of* stewardship instead of exploitation; of fostering consensus instead of competition; of spiritual expression instead of a lust for recognition and influence; of mentoring rather than directing. Elderhood is wisdom in an active state utilized on behalf of others. Older men and women express elder like behavior by taking the journey that leads them to a fourfold balance intellectually, emotionally, physically and spiritually. This fourfold balance places emphasis on all four of these aspects of being. Elders are as concerned with their physical health as they are with their spiritual status. They know they are still learning and have a willingness to show who they are emotionally.

An elder is a sage, not only wise but also experienced and, therefore, an elder is advanced in years. It takes a long time to gain the experience needed to develop elder wisdom which is deeper, tested and built on decades of learning from their mistakes.

Elders have been, throughout history, people who celebrate life and energize others with their passion and hopefulness. They can more accurately assess their personal strengths and skill because they know their limitations. Elders have their faults but carry themselves well despite the fact that they are human. Elders operate from their heart, their center. A centered person is patient, loving and available to others. Elders are centered and, therefore, can be motivating and invigorating at the spiritual level.

Community, interpersonal cooperation and consensus stir elders because these are expressions of spirit in the world. Elders speak their minds and are generative which to me means they have a life giving energy others can absorb. The generative person facilitates growth and creation: a process begun by God that goes on day after day. The elder is also Earth-friendly in their admiration of creation. The ancient and universal archetypes of the mature person suggest a pride that comes from the conscious care of one's own health, as well as their family and kinship with Earth and its limited resources. A person is operating with elder energy if people are liberated, empowered and healed by their presence.

An example of elder expression is the good grandmother who at once enwraps her children with life assuring warmth and, at the same time, lets them go and grow to become independent and free adults. Another example is the journeyman who mentors the apprentice with goals of sponsorship and advocacy as well as the demonstration of skills. Elders believe the role of adults is to facilitate creativity in the young, not teach the patterns of the past. This often leads to mentoring, and mentoring is time consuming. Elders, therefore have less time to indulge themselves. Elders, in their wisdom, sense that they are caretakers and that their vitality depends on a personal shift from egocentricity to community.

One Elder

Doug was the manager of human resources in a large company. He supervised Ivy, a woman who coordinated benefits for employees. She was known as the "iron lady" because of her stern and aggressive interpersonal style. Those of us who knew the "iron lady" watched her evolution into a more gracious adult as she allowed Doug to influence her. The mere experience of being around Doug caused her to change. One notable day, Doug went to her after she had explained to an employee, rationally but impatiently, how the employee's health insurance didn't cover marriage counseling. Doug said to her, "Ivy, the employee was revealing to you indirectly that he had marital problems. He was looking for information, which you gave him. However, he could have been seeking help."

"Are you saying I should be his marriage counselor?" Ivy responded defensively.

"You are the benefits manager in a department of human resources. You have knowledge about resources that he doesn't have. You could both listen briefly and refer him." Doug said.

"I didn't think of that. I moved too quickly didn't I?" Ivy concluded.

"A person with the knowledge you have can be a wonderful resource," said Doug. "Ivy, each time a person comes to you, try to leave them with a little more than they had when they walked in," Doug said.

Doug is a man who can tap elder energy in himself when needed. Ivy trusted him because she felt safe with Doug. He had his faults but Ivy had worked with him long enough that she had come to believe he was a mentor and not a competitor nor a bureaucrat wanting only to wield his power. Ivy went on to become a very good human resource manager herself. She was stirred by Doug's natural ability to reach into the hearts of other people. Generative people like Doug access a balance of masculine and feminine energies from the human soul and psyche. Generativity is that quality of interpersonal connection that empowers others. If Ivy "grows up" to become elder like herself, it will be in part because she was energized and motivated by Doug.

Spiritual Journey

Because the second half of life is considerably longer today than it ever was in the past, we should ask if this longevity has a purpose. Longer life is a blessing that allows more time to ask questions, more time with family, and more time to play. It leaves more "time to drink wine, to eat bread not by yourself but by some other magic" (Pintauro, 1968, p.15). Spiritual teachers who, down the ages, have taught that our presence here is more than biological, more than coincidental, say that to manifest our true being requires a spiritual journey. Could the extraordinary long lives of people today suggest that our extra time on Earth is to be used to deepen a spiritual journey? Most soulful philosophers teach us that the purpose of living on Earth is to achieve union with our essential nature. Our essential nature is our spirit, the aspect of life that connects us to one another and to the divine. Spirit person Howard Thurman called this nature and the mystery of it, the Luminous Darkness (Thurman, 1965). Both Earth and humankind are healed somewhat every time someone advances on their spiritual journey. We are spiritual beings on the human journey as well as humans on a spiritual journey.

I believe that the crowning expression of a fourfold approach to personal balance that facilitates elder expression is the spiritual one. While possessing psychological, intellectual and physical health is essential to a person's experience of being, being spiritual connects us to all that makes up wholeness: people; Earth; and however you define God or whatever unifying force ties it all together for you. "The human spirit cannot abide the enforced loneliness of isolation. We literally feed on each other; where this nourishment is not available, the human spirit and the human body—both—sicken and die" (Thurman, 1971, p.3). A spiritual life is different than a "religious" life. Belonging to a religion is sectarian and provides people with dogma and practices that structure but it can also separate believers into faith groups.

Spirit is in the soul at the very center of our being where God is found. According to Matthew Fox, a key promoter of the Creation Spirituality tradition and author of *Original Blessing,* spirituality is about the source of life, namely, the spirit. "…there is only one Spirit, one breath, one life, one energy in the universe" (Fox, 1991, p.12). Elderhood is not only wisdom in action but it is spirituality expressed. "Spiritual eldering implies an inner search for God, a self-directed flowering of the spirit that unites all people in a common quest, no matter what their affiliation" (Schachter-Shalomi, 1995, p.39). It is the embracing of our spiritual selves that allows us to move from childhood and adulthood to elderhood. Through the "walk of elder" we recover an ancient tradition of oneness with creation. Ancient elders were often the community's link to the ancestors and thus, to the cosmos. Gandhi said that the only way to find God was to "see Him in His creation and be one with it" (Gandhi, 1984, p.57). Elders make a connection to others and the energy that creates that connection is spirit. We can touch the skin of others physically. We can understand others intellectually. We can feel the joys and sorrows of others emotionally. However, we can only connect to others by flowing in the spirit.

In that the reader will find references to the "soul" in this work, it is useful to define it further here. Firstly, for me the soul is fed by the spirit which is the energy of the Universe. Paradoxically, the soul is closer to God than to the human body of man even though it resides in our bodies.

The 13th Century mystic, Meister Echhart, said "...for the soul is nearer to God than it is to the body which makes us human" (Oxford, 1997, p.303). When our body dies the senses dissolve and the mind drops away. "Consciousness then merges with the 'Clear Light' 'the primordial ground of our absolute nature'" (Schachter, p.172). The "Clear Light" is God and God's creation. The soul then is that aspect of the human that is eternal, that pre-existed the human condition and that returns to creation after death: the afterlife.

The Four Paths

One way of understanding my spirituality is to review what advocates of Creation Spirituality call, the Four Paths. The spiritual journey that embraces Creation Spirituality is a revision of spirituality found in mainline Christianity. Matthew Fox says that the four paths "are signposts, reassurances that we are not traveling alone but with the entire mystical body: the communion of saints and the Creation Spirituality tradition, past, present and future. With this body, the entire movement of Creation Spirituality journeys along a spiral path" (Fox, 1991, pp.18-19). Unlike the human developmental processes described by Erik Erikson, Robert Bly, Angeles Arrien, Robert Moore and Douglas Gillette that are discussed in Chapter Six, following the four paths is spiral, not linear. Elder expression can deepen as a man or woman ventures onto their spiritual journey. I stated above that the journey into elderhood is a spiritual pathway. We can understand this in one way by overlaying the elder's journey with the four paths of Creation Spirituality.

The first of the four paths is the *Via Positiva*: a way of affirmation, awe and revelry. The person who is elder like is in awe of creation. These special older people are out of the rat race and free once again to celebrate life. This is the essence of the *Via Positiva*. Like they did as a child, elders following this path once again befriend creation. It leads to the elder role of earthkeeper. The older person who befriends creation knows:

> The earth is not a dead body, but is inhabited by a spirit that is life and soul. All created things, minerals included, draw their strength from the earth spirit. The spirit is life, it is nourished by the stars: and it gives nourishment to

all the living things it shelters in its womb. Through the spirit received from on high, the earth hatches the minerals in her womb as the mother her unborn child. (Valentinus, 2004)

The *Via Negativa*, a way of letting go, of emptying and letting pain strip us of our cover-ups, is the second path. The elder does not kid herself about her perfection, wisdom or personal strength. The humility that is elder expression comes in large part from the elder's understanding and acceptance without guilt of their imperfection, naiveté and weaknesses. Speaking like an elder the poet Rumi said,

> When I am sad, I am radiant
> When I am broken, content
> And when I am tranquil and silent as the earth
> My cries like thunder tremble heaven (Harvey, 1994, p.99).

The elder, therefore, is able to "let go and let God". This is the essence of the *Via Negativa*. James Hillman suggests that older persons need to shift from a focus on "lasting" to an acceptance of "leaving". "The move from lasting to leaving changes our basic attitude from holding on to letting go" (Hillman, 1999, p.53). It is not us who are leaving, however. It is a set of assumptions and attitudes that were useful in our youth. These beliefs are no longer as functional as they were in our earlier years.

The *Via Creativa* is the third path. It is a way of personal creativity and an unfolding of a continuing creation. The way we will see the elder in Chapter Four is as people who are once again able to be creative and playful. At the same time they are generative and in this nurturing energy co-create with God. Elders continue to grow as well as facilitate the growth of the people they serve. In our elder generativity we are cocreative with God and in our imaginative output we trust our images enough to birth them.

The *Via Transformativa*, a way of compassion and social justice, is the fourth path. In the *Via Transformativa* is found the drive to serve. One of the great questions the aspiring elder must ask is not "What am I doing here?" but "Who am I here for?" This is reflective of the fourth path. The challenge for the older person, however, is differentiating between the hero and the wise person. The hero can fight for justice and be on the path of the *Via Transformativa*. "As ripened adults, we have much to contribute to the world seemingly gone mad. But we can't help the world if we ourselves are driven. We need to cultivate not just *doing*, but a quality of *being*: at peace in Sabbath time" (Leder, 1997, p.xiv). The wise can transform within a state of being, come home and become accessible to the young.

Facilitator of Journey

The elder can facilitate the march of other people down their spiritual path. They do this in part by modeling soulful expression both among people and in relationship to Earth. Buddhists, believing that spiritual masters are enlightened beings, sometimes say that attaining liberation from the ego and its fear-induced life style, that is, to reach enlightenment, is only possible by following a spiritual model—the master. For me, a spiritual master would be a person who, in the eyes of their disciples, expresses elder-like behaviors. One Buddhist priest said about the influence of his master on the disciple's pathway, "The sun's rays fall everywhere uniformly, but only where they are focused through a magnifying glass can they set dry grass afire" (Rinpoche, 1993, p.136). The master is the disciple's magnifying glass.

Buddhists believe that the adoration of their master, their teacher, brings them closer to *nirvana*: the extinguishing of worldly desires and attachments so that a union with the Creator is possible. Therefore, the disciple's admiration is largely an affirmation, an unconscious attempt to make the spiritual teacher an elder. When the disciple's devotion to the master brings the disciple to the point where they literally believe the master to be nothing less than the Buddha, the disciple is ready to become a master as well. In this way the master, is "holding the spiritual container" for the disciple.

The concept of a spiritual guide like the Buddhist master has all but disappeared in the West. Westerner naiveté about gurus and elders of other world traditions leads some to believe that eldering means seeking out a high mountain cave and becoming contemplative with limited human contact like the sannyasin in Hindu tradition. The fascination some have with sages around the world suggests an image of elder as reclusive. Even Buddhists, however, in their irrational admiration of spiritual teachers, assume the elder in their life is going to be accessible. What good is an inaccessible teacher?

In the mystical Islamic tradition called the Sufi, an elder is expected to prove one's love for humanity in part by interacting with people and being accessible to them. The Sufis don't believe that their spiritual teachers are perfect in the way Buddhists do, but they expect the teacher to show "mother-spirit, the father-spirit, the brother-spirit, the child-spirit, the friend-spirit...an ever tolerant nature...compassion [and a] thorough understanding of human nature" (Khan, 1964, p.77). These are still pretty classy credentials, however, especially for people of the West. Two keys to an elder's credibility whether it is in a Western, Buddhist or Sufi tradition are first, the elder's willingness to be available to share wisdom and secondly, the trust of the persons who would receive the wisdom.

It is the synergy with one's student that completes the teacher.

Blessing by Elders

When my oldest son reached the age of 18 years, I felt a need to release him. I had been aware only at an intellectual level that I would need to let him go someday. It felt like he was ready not so much to be an adult but rather to be honored as a boy who was ready to consider adulthood. My wife and I planned a ceremony that would bless our son and show our respect for his individuality.

On the day of his "blessing ceremony", we gathered in our home with all our children. We played music we thought conveyed the feeling of honor and love. My wife and I wore clothes that my son would consider unique and special for his day. Each of the six of us, in turn, told our eldest son and brother what we appreciated about him, his uniqueness and his beauty. Each of us closed our brief remarks with a spontaneous hug. As the oldest member of our nuclear family, I acted as the family's representative and presented my son with a gift that symbolized his maturity and the family's confidence that he was becoming a man. His name is Caleb but he had created a fantasy name for himself, Draxx. Caleb is an avid reader of myth and loves J.R.R. Tolkein. Our gift to him was a full size sword of the kind warriors in Tolkein's stories might carry. We had the name, Draxx, engraved on the blade. Caleb breathlessly took the sword from my hands and held it like it was a delicate piece of art. He was speechless but we all knew we had hit pay dirt with that sword.

With each of our five children, my wife and I have been drawn to ceremonially let each child go and to encourage his or her adulthood with a ceremony like Caleb's. Our children have selected my wife and I as elders of their family — their nuclear family. They have also embraced other special, trustworthy adults in our extended family as elders. The blessing ceremony was an endorsement, an affirmation of each child that a trusted elder is capable of offering. As my children grow they have found other older people they trust. They have initiated these people into the role of elder by giving them their trust.

The people in the community who bless others include ministers, coaches, teachers and some employers. If we observe closely, the "blessing", the affirmation that these trusted elders offer, has at least five parts:
- Touch
- Special words
- An expression of appreciation to the ones being blessed
- Referencing for the ones being blessed a dream or special future
- An active commitment to the ones being blessed to help them realize their future, their dream (Smalley, 1990)

We can affirm people through this process of unconditional positive regard. This affirmation plays a role in the growth of those being blessed. We can see this in ceremonies like the offering of a crown in croning ceremonies or in the laying on of the sword in the bestowing of knighthood. The one being blessed is honored and is believed to have moved from one spiritual realm to another one. They grow. They are initiated. The blessing is usually performed by an older person who is respected by the community. The blessing is offered in sacred space — holy ground created when people are seen and heard, recognized, admired and affirmed by another. If the person being blessed is ready emotionally, intellectually, physically and spiritually, the affirmation can change a person's life forever.

The process of blessing which is like initiation has four aspects: 1. A community's endorsement, 2. Sacred space, 3. An elder's affirmation and 4. Readiness and absorption of the blessing by the one being blessed. First we are held by the love of our family and friends. Then sacred space forms. As we will see more and more below, the spokesperson in a community blessing is often a respected, older person. Finally, the blessing can only take if the one blessed is open to and willing to accept the offer.

A Father's Blessing

My father gave me a shotgun when I turned 13. He occasionally had taken me pheasant, duck and pigeon hunting. Giving me the gun was his best try at saying to me, "You are becoming a man". The act of presenting me with the shotgun had the potential of blessing. He didn't initiate me into knowing about the danger of holding a loaded gun or honor my fear of the gun but, nevertheless, it was a "laying on of hands". He might better have taken me aside, listened to my questions and made of the moment a more memorable experience. Men have yearned for fathers who could take us by the arm and lead us into the world of other men. The community's endorsement came from other male hunters who showed me deference because I carried a gun. Sacred space was created, however, by my father's focus on me, by his show of love for me with the gift and the offering to me of the affirmation. My father attempted to bless me by trusting me with the responsibility of owning a shotgun. The gun remains today one of my most treasured possessions even though I never chose to become a hunter as an adult. When my youngest son, Jeremy, reached 21, I presented the shotgun to him. This was one of the finest moments Jeremy and I have ever experienced together.

Initiation

The philosopher and mythologist Joseph Campbell, psychologist Erik Erikson, educator Jean Piaget and others have proposed schematics for stages of growth, of human development. An aspect of growth is the process of initiation where a person moves through a stage of development as a result of a focused ceremony. Initiation can be a fundamental element of movement from a less mature stage of development to the next stage. Initiation is also a ceremonial admission into a group or society. For the initiate, the ceremony is the kick off to a new beginning, an introduction. It requires instruction by those sponsoring the initiate in the fundamentals or principles of the new group or society.

In the United States, men's and women's gatherings have experimented with initiation rituals for a number of decades now. Through organized weekend meetings or by building small communities in ongoing men's groups, men have been looking for something they missed in the course of growing up. The sponsors of these gatherings and workshops seek to create an environment that facilitates healing and personal growth through the use of small group exercises, drumming and mock experiences that facilitate grieving and initiation rituals copied from traditions including African and Native American. They try to replace the elements of initiation the men missed as they were growing up. In croning ceremonies the "talking circle" is often the essence of the gathering. Whoever holds the talking stick has the floor. When she speaks no one interrupts. When the woman talking finishes, she passes to anyone seeking to speak.

Anthropologist Arnold Van Gennep studied the ceremonies of various cultures that accompanied passages from one part of a person's life to another. He coined the phrase "rites of passage". These rites, he said, honored the reality that "life itself means to separate and to be reunited, to change form and... to die and to be reborn... And there are always new thresholds to cross: the thresholds of summer and winter, of a season or a year, of a month or a night; the thresholds of birth, adolescence, maturity, and old age; the threshold of death..." (Gennep, 1960, p.50).

The fourth element of blessing mentioned above, the hunger and readiness of the initiate, is evident at men's initiation weekends and in crone gatherings because these events are created to appeal to people interested in personal growth. The two elements of blessing that usually aren't present in North America, however, are true community and its representative elder. The weekend gatherings I have attended provided a newly formed, temporary community with an individual or individuals assigned the role of "elder for the weekend" or what is called in some men's organizations, the ritual elder. Community can't be created in a weekend, however. The communities that know a person well enough to celebrate his or her passages from one developmental level to another take years to form. They include family, church and sometimes hometown neighborhoods. Others are fraternal lodges, professional associations and labor organizations. In each of these communities older persons who have built personal credibility over an extended period of time are often shown extraordinary deference and are asked to represent the community to younger initiates. The ritual elder of weekend workshops I have taken is only a symbol of this community endorsed elder. Elders of older cultures naturally rose to this role as they grew into credibility. They were not created artificially.

Many have found that the family is the best community in which to grow through the stages of life. Some mothers and fathers understand the importance of initiation and understand what Prophet Kahlil Gibran said in *The Prophet*:

> Your children are not your children. They are the sons and daughters Of life's longing for itself. They come through you but not from you. And though they are with you yet they belong not to you... You are the bows from which your children as living arrows are sent forth. Let your bending in the Archer's hand be for gladness; For even as He loves the arrow that flies, so He loves also the bow that is stable (Gibran, 1951, p.18).

Not all parents have the ability, knowledge and the passion for facilitating their children's growth and many people in North America lack a church community. A neighborhood can keep changing as new families move in and out. In today's fast changing world, people don't put down many roots. Professional associations often lack depth and there has been a decreasing membership in fraternal organizations. College fraternities and sororities don't usually get to know each member well enough to qualify, as a body of people, who understand personal needs for advocacy and initiation in the process of growing up.

By the time I met my wife, she and I had formed separate communities of friends that knew and loved us. Both my family and my personal friends endorsed my marriage to Linda. They wanted for me the joy and stability marriage would bring. To bestow a blessing, we selected a priest because my wife is Catholic. He had the credentials to marry us but he was not a member of my community. The people who spoke for our community and who were intimate enough with my wife and me were our parents. They were the elders in this ceremony. They were the people most passionately involved with us. To see us, hear us and release us. Our parents knew of our need for their endorsement and their sponsorship of our growth. My parents saw a role for themselves in our marriage ceremony, but they didn't think of themselves as facilitators of an initiation. For this reason we engaged a professional initiator in the person of the priest.

Elderhood

A few years ago, a good friend said to me, "You have no choice about it, you are an elder." He was reacting to my reluctance to accept leadership in a spiritual community of which he and I were co-founders. I wanted to simply participate in the group and not be burdened with the role of board member. He saw that the group was in need of leadership and he recognized my ability to facilitate groups. He knew I operated a successful business. Joseph Campbell wrote, "The first requirement of any society is that its adult membership should realize and represent the fact it is they who constitute its life and being... [and to] establish in the [young] a system of sentiments that will be appropriate to the society in which he is to live, and on which that society itself must depend for its existence." (Campbell, 1972, p.46). Campbell wanted certain adults to move from adulthood to elderhood and in this way these elders could embrace the society and hold the sacred container.

The elder, unlike the elderly, know they owe advocacy to young people. I have redefined the word elderly. The elderly complain about aging or spend their retirement separating themselves from the young. Elders continue to deepen their experience of living. The elderly remain angry about experiences that hurt them throughout their life. They have not yet forgiven. The elder attempts to forgive. While the young move from "obscurity into prominence, from present to future, the elder moves back home, into the past, and toward the deeper and more fundamental strata of human experience." (Chinen, 1989, pp.150-151). The elderly don't celebrate life in the way the elder does. They are just trying to get through it. What many of us are hungering for is a quality in older people called elderhood. Rabbi Zalman Schachter-Shalomi approached this idea by describing elderhood as a "state of consciousness that arises in the context of physiological aging... [where] the psyche issues a call for us to engage in life completion, a process that involves specific tasks, such as coming to terms with our mortality, healing our relationships, enjoying our achievements and leaving a legacy for the future." (Schachter-Shalomi, pp.16-17). The elderly resist the call to engage in the personal work necessary to growing into elderhood. The resistance results both from immaturity in adulthood and a submission to the weight of bias toward the old.

To be absolutely clear about the difference between elder and elderly we need to further assess the derivation of the word, elder. In the Christian church the term "elder" was copied from the ancient Israelites. The Hebrew Scriptures tells of the elders appointed by Moses to assist him in the task of community management. Elders in the Mormon Church are nearly all men age 20 and over no matter their level of involvement in the church. The Presbyterians in the 16th Century referred to both "teaching elders" and "ruling elders". They were laymen chosen by the congregation to assist the minister in the governing of the church. The elders in religious traditions like these were not necessarily elder like in the way I emulate the role of elder in this book.

Elders who manage churches have usually been men, men with an interest in management and service. Although the church elder may also be elder like, this is coincidental. The one thing these men have in common with the archetype of elder is that they are often selected from the community of persons whom they serve. Generative elders, people who can't resist being a resource to others, become elders only after they are endorsed by others who find them to be accessible, patient and wise celebrants of life.

Elders are more balanced than the elderly. They aren't necessarily holy people, however. The elder in America is going to look quite American. They probably won't look to us like a shaman or priestess. If an elder feels like a shaman or priestess to those who benefit from their wisdom, fine. But, American elders may dress conservatively or old fashioned. They may, like the older people around them, drive too slow, golf a lot, garden or enjoy classes taught at the local senior center. What makes them different is the need those around them feel to be in their presence. The treasure that elders bring is the potential liberation of the archetypal energies within him or her that brings them to be a balanced, mature and responsive older person. An elder is a spokesperson for the community.

To understand the bias toward aging in the West is to understand in part why only a few older people are willing to embrace the role of elder. This discomfort with being old goes way back in American history. Consider these words by Henry David Thoreau.

> Age is no better, hardly so well, qualified for an instructor as youth, for it has not profited so much as it has lost.

> One may almost doubt if the wisest man has leaved anything of absolute value by living. Practically, the old have no very important advice to give the young, their own experience has been so partial...and they are only less young than they were. I have lived some thirty years on this planet, and I have yet to hear the first syllable of valuable or even earnest advice from my seniors" (Thoreau, 1980, p.8).

Thoreau may have been looking too hard for advice and less for the healing energy of a loving elder. Elder advice can be valuable but not as powerful as the force of their gentle presence. Nevertheless, it is likely that this poet seldom came across older people who were brave enough to step up and mentor, pass on wisdom, develop a partnership with nature or offer blessing (I will develop the idea of partnership with nature below).

The archetypal elder has been the same force in most cultures over most all of time. An archetype is an ancient model for a role that has survived time. I referred to the archetypal elder within in my first book when discussing the energy from the psyche that energizes those who express elderhood. Just as the instincts seem to account for recurrent behavior patterns in humankind, so the archetypes seem to account for recurrent psychic patterns. Psychic patterns are expressions of the psyche. The psyche is all of the human being, which is not physical or spiritual. The psyche includes the conscious and unconscious elements of the human personality. When a person taps the energy of the elder within, these qualities of elderhood are available to them:

- balance in our expression of intellect, spirit, body and heart
- knowledge of our faults, our shadow
- an expression of self principally from our center, our soul
- patience and a desire to be available to others
- an awareness of our personal strength
- a sage like love for consensus and community
- wisdom
- a passion for Earth and its survival
- generativity
- stewardship energy of Earth, of people

- a desire to take care of ourselves and take pride in our good health
- knowledge that we are caretakers whose vitality depends on a personal shift from self to community
- a personal force that empowers others when they are in our presence.
- a hunger to introduce the meaning of life to the young

My Search

In the early part of 1990, I turned 50 years old. In February of that year, I had ventured with sixty other people to a spiritual retreat on a Pacific island. We were housed in rustic facilities at a retreat center set in a jungle. Just across the road was the ocean. Having lived on the Pacific coast of the USA for most of my life, I was acquainted with the ocean. But I had not, until then, been on a relatively small body of land surrounded by the great body of water. The island was volcanic. Within two miles of our location, a flow of molten lava was pushing unyieldingly down the mountainside towards the sea. I was surrounded for ten days with unfamiliar flora, fragrances completely new to me, and animal and insect life that intimidated me. It was in this place, at this time, that I made a leap in my spiritual journey. I believe that I needed isolation in a place where the energy of Earth was overwhelming so that I might discover my reason for being, a key dimension of the spiritual journey.

It wasn't a curiosity about my reason for being, however, that moved me to begin this journey. I had, for a number of years, been feeling empty, and I lacked depth. I had very little spark to get me going each day. The emptiness inside me needed filling. I had a wonderful wife and family, professional success and fair health, but the emptiness was overwhelming. I sensed that there was more. What I was experiencing was a primal feeling of separation from a place deep within me—my soul. My first step on my pathway to elderhood was to confront the separation. What began that week as I ended midlife and entered the second half of life was a conversion to a belief in a purpose. One way I know that God exists is my belief that we are in this life for a purpose. Either we are here, in this existence, for some reason, or we pass through life simply by accident. I decided I was here for a purpose. I began addressing life from my heart, the doorway to the soul. I began questioning my shadow expressions and the damage I did when shadow energy ran my day. I started to shift away from only "doing" toward a contemplative experience of "being". Elders, I came to learn, are on a spiritual journey that can for some even feel involuntary. I began a move from adulthood into elderhood.

From my anecdotal research I have come to know that the average person has met only a few elder like people. The elders either have gone underground or are simply few in number. As my hunger to meet them grew, in 1995 I began a search for those who expressed elderhood. In my wallet, I carried a card that describes an elder. I carry it with me yet today. Elders, I speculated on the card:

- Are seasoned, and a source of life-giving energy
- Know their limitations and are skillful
- Have an unconquerable spirit
- Are knowledgeable, aware and filled with insight
- Are intuitive, passionate, spiritual and sensuous

I began asking people if they knew a person of wisdom. I told people I was seeking out elders so that I could interview them and I read the card out loud to them. In the past few years I have found my way to increasing numbers of people who express elder like behaviors. How important these people are! They are a resource for young people. None of them is a Mahatma Gandhi, a Mother Theresa, Winston Churchill, Florence Nightingale or a Martin Luther King Jr. Few of them have needed to risk their life for a cause. Few of them have written a book or gained media attention in any way. Their greatness stems from their willingness to share their wisdom and help heal, to express their humor and their soulful spirit.

The elders I have met so far have had two things in common: they were in touch with their spiritual life and they were imperfect. They were as close to having a fourfold balance of psychological, physical, spiritual and intellectual expression as anyone I have met and yet they all had historical and ongoing personal problems that could, at anytime, interfere in their balance. They all struck me as intelligent and emotionally expressive people. Wise people feel that way. They varied in levels of intelligence. What was true to all is that they were patient, often at peace with themselves and tolerant of others. They were generative, loving people in whose presence I felt empowered. Paradoxically, it was increasingly inaccurate to call them elders. They were very often elder like but to say they are elders is difficult. They don't call themselves elders. They are good examples of adults who are moving into elderhood but they are still human. Sometimes I place elderhood too high among human goals. It is a way of being I aspire to and, too often I forget that anyone can have elder qualities and yet still live out of their shadow, still sometimes be immature.

To address life from the center, the spirit, does not mean a person needs to be perfect. The elder like people we know are not gods. Our reverence for them may suggest to the reader that they are godlike when, in fact, they are wonderfully human. They admit openly that they struggle with the challenges of the ego, their humanness. Three whom I have met are recovering alcoholics. Some of them were workaholics. Some still drink too much. One man declared to me that his manner is too often childlike and he knows he doesn't fit many people's view of a grown-up. And another admits that her stressful approach to life has caused her significant health problems. My search surfaced only a few people initially. Why is it so difficult to find elders in the Western world?

Elders and the Aged Lose Credibility

There is a hunger among people for mentors. This hunger dates back to the time when extended family began to disintegrate. Women today have an average of about two children in their lifetime. Before 1860, families consisted of over five people. This was primarily a nuclear family with an occasional grandparent. The pre-industrial era village contained numerous extended family members (Demos, 1986, p.5). The master craftsmen and other elders such as aunts and uncles and friends of the extended family left their agrarian home about 200 years ago. They went away to work in the cities to feed their families. The work they went to do often lacked meaning. It provided an income but it removed them from Earth. It made subsistence possible and yet was focused on earning wages. Life and livelihood can be "about living in depth, living with meaning, purpose, joy, and a sense of contributing to the greater community" (Fox, 1994, p.2). Elderhood includes a confidence in "good work". Doing good work means doing what we have an inner calling to do. We want to do this kind of work no matter the wages.

In the USA our assumptions about home, work, women and women's relationship to productivity changed permanently by the 19th Century. "The earliest factories were actually the homes of agricultural workers who began producing textiles, iron, glass and other commodities...Women had worked alongside men even at the forges...and the textile industry in particular had always depended on women" (Rich, 1976, p.25). Gradually younger women were driven into the mills just like the men. This move, this enclosure of men and women away from the home, began the destruction of Earth that is so apparent today. The pride of the elders, the spirit and joy of the elders, and the husbandry by the elders began to suffer when the men and women left home. Another historical event added to the diminution of the elders: the immigration from Europe to America.

An uncontrolled movement of people from all world cultures into the United States occurred in the 19th Century. It was the young and hardy that took on this adventure. Most of the older people remained in their native countries. The American culture from about 1900 on was made up of the children of immigrants. Absent were the elders because they were still in their home country. The offspring of the immigrants were forced to create a culture based largely on their observation of their peers, who offered more practical models than those of the few elders who did immigrate. The past of the older people was inaccessible to them. The ancestors of some of the world's primitive cultures like the Eskimos, for example, who historically had come from an Oriental culture in the Old World, also lacked the knowledge and depth and variety of experience needed to thrive in the New World. Most of the Eskimo elders remained in their natural surroundings in Asia.

The founding "fathers" in this country were in fact "founding sons, rebellious sons, refugees from patriarchal gerontocracy. They had run from the stifling tradition of being monitored by the repulsive, chiding, gossiping elders in claustrophobic villages" (Gutmann, 1994, p.9). Industrialization and the breakup of the extended family and immigration separated old men and women from the young. In pre-modern times, before the 18th Century, the young discovered adulthood by being in close proximity to parents and older people who were living in the same village. Older people did not need to be balanced and devoted elders to model accessibility. The mere fact that they were not mobile, remained in the community and had long lives meant that they could be a resource to the young. Some of the older people exhibited elder like behavior but all older people, mature or not, left behind a pathway for the young to assess.

In America today, old people are denigrated. In my experience many find people over 60 years of age to be noxious, in their way, bothersome, weak and lacking in intelligence. The distance we feel between older people and the young is, however, not a uniquely Western problem. Retiring older people, in turn, try to drown out any positive intuition we might have about aging through diversions such as travel, entertainment, alcohol abuse and other obsessive habits. Old people remind us of our mortality. Our judgment in the West is that death is a mistake and we try to avoid it as long as possible. Embracing death as a part of life, however, is guaranteed to deepen a person's appreciation of life. Elders have a "detached concern with life...in the face of death itself," according to psychologist Eric Erikson. (Erikson, 1986, pp.37-38). Our denigration of older people is more an expression of our fear of aging than a statement about the value of older people.

Sigmund Freud theorized that two forces drive human experience: *libido*, the life instinct and *thanatos*, the death instinct. Freud believed life included a struggle between these two forces. "*Libido* surges with vitality, seeking pleasure and continuity of experience. *Thanatos* longs to return to an inanimate state of quiescence devoid of all striving and conflict" (Schachter-Shalomi, p.83). In *The Prophet* Gibran wrote, "Your fear of death is but the trembling of the shepherd when he stands before the King whose hand is to be laid upon him in honor. Is the shepherd not joyful beneath his trembling that he shall wear the mark of the King? Yet is he not more mindful of his trembling?" (Gibran, p.71). When we access the death instinct we can be energized in a way that is comparable to the charge we get from *libido*. If we accept our mortality we are more inclined to celebrate the time we have left on Earth and get the most out of the present moment.

When Westerners, especially those who are male, first consider the *libido* and its drives, they assume with trembling that the *libido* begins to die in the second half of life. It is at this time, they muse, that the completing and contemplative instincts of thanatos replace the *libido*. This brought up a problem for me, however: a number of large, stressful and action-oriented challenges came into my life when I passed the age of 50. I shifted from my professional occupation into an energetic and creative occupation with elderhood and the research that went into it. I had to let go of my children as they matured and moved into their adult lives. My wife took off professionally and at age 50, she was as vigorous and passionate about her work as I had been in my thirties. While I was gradually resting into a quieter and less aggressive style of living, I was also charged with new passions, new relationships, a "new" wife and new activities that came with these new charges. My *libido* was calmed in some ways but was elevated in others. At 50, I was beginning to be drawn by the siren call of *thanatos*, but it could be many years, I judged, before contemplation, reminiscing, meditation, listening and quiet days of minimal anxiety would be mine.

The way we think about elders is lost in how we view the elderly. Our fear of death and our consequent desire to stay young and stay around young people gets in the way of seeking out elders. Our language overflows with words and phrases we use to separate ourselves from old people: "relic of the past, old relic, out-of-date, not-with-it, old fossil, obsolete, over-the-hill, old fogey, old codger, old crock, crotchety, decrepit, doddering, gray beard, senile, outmoded, little old man/lady, wizened, wrinkled, superannuated, archaic, second childhood, dotage, past their prime, having one foot in the grave, antiquated, toothless, old biddy" (Larue, 1992, p.39). When the United States was formed in 1776, our founders turned to the young for energy and their hunger for individual expression. The "New Americans" wanted to avoid the mistakes and excesses that had reduced the Mother Country into an old, wrinkled, withered, worn-out hag! Interesting it was, however, that we chose the bald eagle as our national bird. One of a young man's fears is growing bald as he ages. If this means some ambivalence prevailed, it probably resulted from the young Americans' wish that the old were more dependable, more accessible and interested in mentoring the young.

The young Americans of the 18th Century displayed "uneasiness with decorum, gentility and the propriety one expects from old people" (Archenbaum, 1986, p.20). A fear of old age and old people was rampant among them. By the end of the 19th Century historian Frederick Turner was appealing to Americans to cherish one's youth. "The older they grow, the more they must reverence the dreams of their youth,"he said. (Mathews, 1951, p.1793).

The Puritans, however, had seen in old people the image of God..."and when His majesty and eternity are set forth in Scripture, it is with white hair" (Turner, 1962, p.339). These early Americans saw the old as standing on the boundary between the "natural and unnatural worlds." The assumption made in pre-modern times even in North America was that the old were wiser because of accumulated experience. In communities where literacy was less common, it was the older people who provided not only wisdom but also a connection to the past. Their memory was the unrecorded history of the people.

"Though your infirmities be never so many and great, you have peculiar honor that is twisted with your infirmity, for it is called the Crown of Age" (Demos,p.143). The old were expected to be dignified in that they wore the Crown of Old Age. This led, incidentally, to the expectation that they would live with restraint. A minister of the 18th Century wrote that the old were "expected to be sober, grave, temperate, sound in faith, charity and patience... They were to be always a living example of the good old way for the public" (Fischer, 1978, p.68). So, not only were the old respected but also they apparently had to work at maintaining that respect. There was an assumption in the community, shared by older people, that being old earned a person a heightened level of respect. In those days it was seldom questioned whether an old person was truly wise. When the old were fewer in number, perhaps it was easier to value them as a resource. "In the world of high fertility and high mortality, where the population was very young and the odds against surviving to a ripe old age were great, respect for age was enhanced by its comparative rarity" (Fischer, p.68).

The Status of the Old

There are other factors that affect the status of old people in a culture. The foremost for males has been property ownership. The influence of the landed citizen has been significant ever since people stopped their nomadic wandering and held onto "things". Two of the most energetic classes of people in American history, however, were the pioneer and the entrepreneur. These two risk-takers were capable of confronting new horizons without the wise old people to guide them. In the New World, young people with new ideas and lots of energy accomplished a great deal on their own. The pioneers found their own land. They had less need for inherited land and, therefore, were less influenced by the older people from whom they might inherit land. The entrepreneur built businesses and accumulated wealth in a community of young and hardy people. The old people who owned land had been left behind.

The next most significant factor determining the status of old people after possession of land is the possession of strategic knowledge. To be "strategic" the knowledge would need to be applicable, for example, in the management of a person's economy, the raising of children or in the maintenance of their health. The old people who immigrated were a resource in their homeland "strategically" but much less in the New World. Another factor determining status has always been the predominant modes and styles of economic productivity (Fischer, p.39). Once again, the old in the New World were less skilled because what they had learned about economy and survival was in another, older culture.

Before the Industrial Era, families were clustered closely together. In the 17th Century the village commons were the primary social units of England. In this system the majority of people, the peasantry at least, comprised a village community of shareholders who utilized the majority of the land on a collective basis. By the 18th Century, millions of craftspeople and artisans in England and throughout Europe were beginning to see the "degradation of their labor and the undermining of their families through the displacement of handicrafts by machines" (Kimbrell, 1995, p.35). The era of machines drew the men away from the village commons and into the new way of life that began the breakdown of the extended family. Old men could not compete for the new industrial jobs. Respect for them by younger men, therefore, began to wane. So, the fourth factor of status, an ethic of mutual dependence, began to loose its potency. The older people became less and less necessary to the survival of the family.

Yet another factor of significance is the importance of received traditions, especially religious ones. Received tradition could be defined as the inherited transmission, from generation to generation, of customs, practices and knowledge. (Demos, p.174) Initiation, discussed earlier in this chapter, is a ceremonial admission into a group or society. Of the four elements of initiation (i.e., community, sacred space, the elder, readiness of initiate) the elder's blessing was an example of a person offering and another receiving tradition. What has happened in modern times is that elders have become less visible and ritual initiation has occurred less often. Tradition is not being "received" as readily as it was in pre-industrial times.

Survival of the Fittest

When in colonial America the older citizen was occasionally appreciated it facilitated continuity, stability, permanence and order in the society. The privileges of old age were apparent in the arrangement of permanent seating in many of the colonial meetinghouses. These community halls were used regularly and were a core aspect of maintaining a sense of community in early America. But, one by one, the governing committees of the meetinghouses changed the seating arrangements. The change began in the late 18th Century and it only took a generation to complete the transition. Rather than assigning seats by age and respect, the committees sold the seats to the highest bidder. The shift from a "pluralistic system of stratification to a unitary system" was based largely on wealth. (Fischer, p.79) A stratified society with the old highly represented at the top was changing.

Adam Smith's *Wealth of Nations* was published in 1776. Smith's philosophy laid the foundation for the free-market doctrine. Smith taught that society could become wealthy by following your self-interest and honoring the laws of supply and demand. In 1859 came Charles Darwin's *Origin of Species* whose dictate was that the strongest and most fit survived in the evolution of all species. Men and women of the industrial era read Darwin to suggest that survival at any price was a natural behavior in the market place. This also suggested that the youngest, richest and most competitive should be preeminent. Around 1800, the authority of age began to be undermined and at the same time the direction of age bias began to be reversed. The doctrine of profit and the ethic of competition were new and unique to Western societies.

People began to move toward the cities and away from the village community of elders, craftsmen and fellow farmers on common land.

Joint work and shared roles in farming and craftsmanship waned in favor of the more competitive world of industrial production (Kimbrell, p.237). Men were becoming a collection of competitors for scarce jobs. The change in older people's relationship to younger was becoming apparent. Older men and women stopped seeing themselves as responsible for teaching and mentoring the young. The young were seen as a threat. The young were becoming more capable of taking over the jobs and they lost respect for the older and less competitive men. Older women remained in the village community longer than the men but they increasingly felt that they were alone as educator for the young. The older men began to loose self-respect as the young men moved into the industrialized world and rejected the older men as incapable of preparing them for the workplace.

In ancient Eastern philosophy such as that found in India, the final and highest stage of life was what the Hindu calls the *sannyasan ashrama*. The final stage began at age 75, when a man left his property and family and lived in poverty with a commitment to self-realization and service to society. In China, Taoism taught that in old age males are set free from the prison of their possessions. The Taoist felt that a person is thus promoted to the rank of living spirit. Although modern people of India and China are questioning the utility of these ancient philosophies, it was primarily Western males who led the way off the land, out of the soul and into the world of competition for wealth that, in a twist of fate, has robbed men and women of independence, security, liberty and birthrights.

The movement away from family and the land was a turning point for male and female gender roles. Women were forced to stay home, watch the children, do the cooking and the washing and generally maintain some connection to the community in which they lived. While some great women including Florence Nightingale, Dorothea Dix and Susan B. Anthony fostered the first feminist movement in the 19th Century, the common woman remained on the land. When women did take jobs in the factories, the family system went into an uproar. A home where women were not always present was "subversive to the patriarchal marriage... the home thus defined had never before existed. It was a creation of the Industrial Revolution" (Rich, p.26). Men and women were away from home while at work. They had to compete for jobs and do work that was meaningless except for the income produced. Work began to mean long hours performing rote tasks away from the family for income earned, not from the sale of crafts but from the sale of a person's time and energy.

Working for money, for gain, is only as old as the 18th Century. The village commons had an economy based on subsistence, handicrafts, barter and the sharing of land. In medieval Christian society, people were condemned for attempting to gain profit from the sale of goods or the loaning of money. The central principle of most pre-modern cultures was gift giving. Anthropologists found that in old cultures financial gain seldom was an "impulse to work under the original native condition" (Polyani,1957, p.270). The Industrial Era concept of working for income alone not only moved people out of the village but also separated them from their reason to celebrate their creativity and survival skills.

The effect of the Industrial Revolution on many other men, women and children was to cause a shifting of the "mute, uneducated, leaderless and now more and more property less common population" towards the new manufacturing areas (Wells, 1920, p.686). There they became a part of the impoverished craftspeople already in place in the growing towns of tacky and unkempt houses. Factories belching black smoke and beginning a devastation to the ecology of two-hundred years were surrounded by the streets of workers' homes, built cheaply, without space rented to the men and women who had moved there from the farms. There were no schools, no churches and nothing that reminded the new residents of creation and God.

Fathers living in the 19th Century began to detach emotionally from their family and were away from home a great deal. This poem written in 1868 depicts the family condition of the family with a father who worked for wages:

>Father is Coming.
>
>The clock is on the stroke of six,
>The father's work is done.
>Sweep up the hearth and tend the fire,
>And put the kettle on.

The wild night-wind is blowing cold.
'Tis dreary crossing o'er the world.
He's crossing o'er the world apace,
He's stronger than the storm;
He does not feel the cold, not he,
His heart, it is warm:
For father's heart is stout and true.,
As ever human bosom knew...
Nay, do not close the shutters child;
For along the land,
The little window looks,
And he can see it shining plain.
I've heard him say he loves to mark
The cheerful firelight through the dark.

Hark! Hark! I hear his footsteps how:
He's through the garden gate.

Run, little Bess, and open the door,
And do not let him wait.
Shout, baby, shout! And clap thy hands,
For father on the threshold stands (Source Unknown).

The mother of the pre-industrial West became more isolated and was left to celebrate family with the working father when he would return from work for short visits lasting only from late supper to an early morning departure.

Elders as Victims of Progress

Great-grandparents living today came from a generation of parents who were among the first victims of the Machine Age, which began around 1850. These people gave up their usable property by leaving the villages and the farms for work in the factories. They lost economic independence by depending on wages. "They lost spiritual independence as their fear of starvation and joblessness made them subservient to their bosses" (Kimbrell, p.39). The soul is alive when one has spiritual independence. Nurturing the soul requires listening to the small voice inside us. The work-a-day world can place a heavy demand on that part of us that is desperate, fearful. This takes us away from our spiritual center and leaves our soul hungry. A person is in a bind vocationally if they can't connect to their spirit:

> In order to meet the definition of success, he must continue to be upwardly mobile, to strive for promotions and to take on greater and greater responsibility. In the process, however, he often has to give up doing that which he once did best, what originally attracted him to his work, and which gave him the deepest satisfactions. As he advances, he will also find it increasingly more difficult to relate to former coworkers and others who were once his friends. If he contents himself with continuing to do the thing he does best and enjoys most and avoids promotion, he may be seen as unsuccessful and may also make his own future vulnerable to those who will pass him by..."(Goldberg, 1976, p.92).

Bias toward women at that time disallowed little more than domestic work and if a woman worked along side men in manufacturing, "Although they developed skills over their careers and helped to train newcomers... they never enjoyed the formal responsibility or the higher status and earnings of supervisors" (Dublin, 1979, p.65). By the late 19th Century, however, women became more and more visible in competition for management roles.

In the race for more promotions, more power and money, I believe people are motivated more by fear and desperation than by satisfaction and qualities that nurture the soul. Men and women who confront life motivated only by competition for power and money are not acting out of their soul. The soul is the "you" that is immortal. The ego, which is not immortal, usually acts out of fear and is inclined to seek power as compensation. Following only the energy of the ego, a person willingly sacrifices intimacy and, thereby lacks wisdom. The soul is a positive, goal directed force that emanates from the center of your being. When a person embraces the nature of elderhood, they exhibit more soulful expression.

The loss of connection to their spirit—their soul—interferes with growth into elderhood.

Because of the bias we have toward older people, I believe the potential elders of the Western world reach the second half of life lacking confidence in their wisdom. Coupled with the resulting lack of pride is a lack of clarity about how to be an elder. Gerald Heard talks about the increasing number of people living to old age as a "new class of the old". They "are utterly untaught, their education is completely neglected, their part is unwritten" (Heard, 1963, p.258). Our community of potential elders has an unprecedented high level of physical health but no models for how to live a full life. "The time at which old age begins is ill defined...nowhere do we find any initiation ceremonies" for a person's entrance into elderhood. (de Beauvoir, 1972, p.50) The quotes above are from writers who are talking about elders in the West. In many cultures outside the Western world, becoming an elder is a natural process for older people.

The potential elders of the new class of the old are living now in an era I call the "Newest Age". The Newest Age is a phenomenon of the last three generations in the West. It has resulted from longer life spans. My grandfather didn't notice it. My father sees it but has no model for it. At age 65, I am entering the Newest Age and I want not only to understand this new opportunity for how to be in an extended life span, but develop a model that can be utilized by others. It begins with a passion for giving back: giving back gifts to the young gained from long life experience so that their pathway through life will be deeper and richer. The Newest Age is potentially an elder renaissance: a time of rebirth of the culture based on a spiritual vision.

Initiation into elderhood begins with a voluntary relinquishment of the personal status and executive authority that we offer to older people. Paradoxically, while we maintain disrespect for aging, we believe that older people attain a level of influence by age alone. "All that is retained is an advisory influence, but even so no specific rulings would be given" (Heard, p.259). This advisory influence is most likely if an older person accepts the role of elder. This automatically implies sharing wisdom with the young.

Mentoring

As mentioned above, myths and tales from pre-modern times contain standards of behavior for elders called archetypes. Allan Chinen says that the archetype of elder found in old stories includes seven tasks that confront people from mid-life forward:

- Dealing with the specter of decline
- Confronting the self and self-reformation
- Shifting from a youthful preoccupation with things to an empathetic understanding of human nature
- Breaking free of personal ambition and dreams, which dominate youth
- Liberating yourself from socially compromising community mores
- Reclaiming wonder and delight in life.
- And, the seventh and most challenging task is said to be "taking the transcendental inspirations of later life and using them to help the next generation" (Chinen, pp.146-147).

Providing counsel and inspiring youth is spiritual stuff! The passion to take the "transcendental inspirations" of later life and use them to help the next generation is called, mentoring. The willingness to mentor the young was doused in many by a fear-driven hunger for survival that was a legacy of the Industrial Era of the 19th Century. In 1818 England workers were trained to work from the age of six, from five in the morning to eight at night. "…he has no relaxation till the ponderous engine stops and then he goes home to get refreshed for the next day; no time for sweet association with his family; they are all alike fatigued and exhausted" (Thompson, 1963, p.201). The potential of older persons as mentors of the young was reduced by our devotion to the "company store" and our distance from the family and the community. A good mentor is a mixture of parent and good friend. Unlike parents and friends, however, mentors are transitional figures who are nevertheless significant in the life of those they serve. They invite a young person into the adult world by acting as guide, teacher, and sponsor. A mentor represents skill, knowledge, virtue and accomplishment but also love.

In early adulthood a young person shifts from being a child to being an adult in a peer relation with other young adults. However, young peers can't model the next level of development toward which the younger man or woman is moving. On the other hand, if the mentor is too parent-like, it is hard for them and the "mentee" to overcome the generational difference and move toward the goal of peer relationship.

The soulful expression of effective mentoring comes as the mentor gives her or his "blessing" to the mentee and honors the dreams of the younger person. The dreams provide a vague sense of what it is like to be true to self in the adult world. The dreams held by the young have the quality of a vision, an imagined possibility that generates excitement and vitality. (Levinson, 1978, p.91) Although examples of a young person's dream surface in mythology and fairy tales, they seldom show up in studies on psychological development. Whether called "the dream", fantasy or a plan for the future, the young are more likely to reach life's goals if the dream has been endorsed, blessed by an older person who is trusted and admired by the young person. A young person has the task of giving their dream meaning and then discovering ways to live it out.

Developing through the stages of human growth is a more complete process if a person structures their life around a dream. If the dream is not satisfied, it may fade away. The person's sense of aliveness and purpose will fade also. As a young adult grows into adulthood, they must separate from their mother and father. They need, therefore, to form relationships with adults who will facilitate their work in realizing the dream. Both a special love relationship and a mentor relationship are of great importance to the task of breaking away from parents and forming an adult life.

Finding mentors is more difficult for men than for women. In premodern times, boys worked side by side with fathers, grandfathers and other extended male family members family. If a young man wanted to seek out other older men, there were craftsmen, clergy and men of other occupations within the community. The smaller communities of the village commons and rural towns were comprised of small gatherings of people mutually dependent upon one another. When a man was ready to exhibit elder-like expression in the form of mentoring, it was easy for the young man to find him. The pre-modern elder was rarely anonymous. Women were accessible and have remained so over the last few centuries more than men. Although it is also true that women elders have become less accessible as they have taken on the high stress activities reserved for men in recent centuries. However, women have a natural inclination to nurture and mentoring is an expression of nurturing energy. "Women have a 'tend and befriend' physiological response; oxytocin—the maternal bonding hormone—increases with stress, which is enhanced by estrogen" (Bolen, 2003, p.100). They have a greater inclination to maintain a connection to people and Earth than men do.

Older women have gathered in groups in North America increasingly since the 1960's. They are increasingly inclined to celebrate their tendency to nurture. The elder women of all cultures have born children and some have served in other ways. Having already brought forth and nurtured the children and their dreams, I feel they have held that it is only in good relationship to themselves, to each other and to Earth that life has any value, meaning or purpose. For too long the voices of women have been silenced. The wisdom of the older women is expressed in their love for the innocents, their respect for the healing gifts of nature and their patience with the unfolding natural rhythms of life. These wise women are good models for the elder role of mentor.

Even though the modern workplace emphasizes teamwork, seldom do workers form mentoring relationships. Even colleges and other schools seem to not foster quality mentoring connections because mentoring is not teaching. Many older person/younger person connections have an aspect of mentorship in them, but true mentoring is not a simple passing on of intelligence. "In a 'good enough' mentoring relationship, the young man feels admiration, respect, appreciation, gratitude and love for a mentor" (Bolen,p.100). A mentor may also teach. He/she may sponsor, using their influence to cause a special opportunity to be revealed to the mentee. A mentor is a host sometimes, introducing the young person to a group, which they want to join or learn about. Mentoring is often like being a guide, reflecting on faulty choices and creative choices. A derivative of the word "prophet" is *nebayoth,* meaning fruitfulness, from Hebrew the verb to germinate… (Fox, 1983a, p.262) and thus to facilitate growth or mentor. Grand parenting and counseling are mentoring functions. To the mentee, the true mentor is a model, an archetype of an elder in the flesh.

The most developmentally crucial role of a mentor is their support for realization of the dream. To love another person is to vibrate with their aspirations, their hopes and their joys. To facilitate the realization of another person's dream is to bless them. To bless someone the mentor needs to share the dream and its possibilities, and feel the charge it causes in a young person's psyche. A mentor must take time to be in tune with the center of another person. People who love take time because they are patient and willing to stand by until the one loved can stand on their own.

It wasn't until Hermann Hesse's *Siddartha* was a grown man that he met his greatest mentor, Vasudeva, the ferryman. The rich man turned buddha, Guatama Siddartha, was seeking enlightenment. From the humble and poor Vasudeva, Siddartha first learned that his mentor was not a teacher. "I am not a learned man, I do not know how to talk or think," said Vasudeva to Siddartha. "I only know how to listen and be devout, otherwise I have learned nothing." Siddartha experienced the joy of having "a listener who could be absorbed in his own life, his own strivings, his own sorrows" (Hesse,1951,p.106). As others with mentors have discovered, Siddartha found that a mentor is trusting and trustworthy, noble, trusts in a Universe larger than himself, is empathetic and affirms life in those for whom they model.

Philosopher Martin Buber wrote in his poem, *The Disciple:*

> The gray hand of the storm lay over both.
> The Master's hair bore a black glow.
> Enveloped and rocked to sleep in dumb suffering,
> Was the face of the disciple, pale and kind.

"The gray hand of the storm" describes the dark passage through fear of the unknown, the unexplored areas of life. Both the "Master" and the "disciple" are affected by the storm, the only certain difference being that the "Master" has been through more of the passages than has the "disciple". Buber continues,

> The way was rocky. Lightning and mountain fire
> Zigzagged around them like trembling branches.
> The boy's step grew weak and ever more timid,
> The old man walked as always, straight and firmly.
>
> The blue eyes gazed dreaming into his own,
> And through the narrow cheeks beat the shame,
> The mouth was set as from repressed weeping,
> The great longing of a child came.

This part has the Master experiencing shame with his mouth "set as from repressed weeping."

Shame is a sense of unworthiness. The older person here feels an obligation to mentor but experiences the fear of not being good enough. And the older person's own longing to be innocent, like a child, rises up. Buber closes with:

> Then the master spoke.
>
> From much wandering
> I took the golden might of the one truth:
> If you can be your own, never be another's.
> And silently the boy walked in the night (Buber, 1967, p.41).

The only thing that the Master assured the boy of was his willingness to be present. The devotion the Master felt to the task of mentoring was so great that the Master felt unworthy, not arrogant. The mentor's wisdom was to assure the boy that the two of them were equals. This devotion is wisdom in action.

Mentoring is a relatively new word. I believe it was created to fill a vacuum formed when the fathers left home. Parents and grandparents are far more than mentors when they act in the fullness of their role. They love like a brother or sister but bring a passion to the relationship no sibling can know. The word mentor was first found in letters written by fathers to their sons. The Oxford English Dictionary found the first use of mentor in the year 1750. A father, separated from his home by the challenge of work in a nearby city, was trying to describe what he missed: raising his children. He used a concept taken from mythology. The teacher whose name was, Mentor, was a friend of Odysseus. His name is now synonymous with a faithful and wise advisor. The act of mentoring, the process that occurs in a generative relationship, did not appear actively in the English language until the middle of the 20th Century.

Mentoring is as close as some people ever get to parenting. In colonial times, parents were central to moral and religious education. They also taught their children basics like reading, writing and math. Fathers approved marriages and apportioned family property. They were in control of the family's property because of the belief in patriarchy, the social organization of family where the father is the supreme head. Exploitation by the patriarch was not one of his most attractive qualities, however, and the concept of patriarchy began to be questioned. The colonial father, however, was "moral overseer, psychologist, and model" and defender of the children against what was believed to be "the emotional, irrational, intellectually inferior and indulgent mother" (Demos, p.44).The Industrial Era changed a lot about what family used to be. The one constant has been the "primary unit". "When the family breaks down...in periods of abrupt transition from one type economy to another ...men may flounder...in these periods, during which the primary unit may again become mother and child, the biological given..." (Mead, 1949, p.192). The obligation and opportunity of fathering and mothering was unquestioned in most pre-modern cultures. People didn't need a word like "mentoring" to describe what was a forgone assumption about the parental role. This was true of many aunts, uncles, craftspeople, ministers and unrelated older villagers as well. Men were the warriors who were to prepare youth for the challenge of being a mature male. Women were the sources of nurture and held the children at the hearth, at the center of the home and the village. They were acting as elders.

Retirement

Older people usually see themselves as being in a state of retirement or wish they were. Although for many retiring is joyful, to retire means to withdraw from career. Our work world structured our time, was a primary source of social connection and provides for most a sense of meaning. Retirement as we imagine it in North America is supposed to offer a life style that is better than the work-a-day world. However, "retiring" means, retreating, to go backward. The elder who is in the third or fourth quarter of their life retreats in a different way. They retreat into contemplative activities where they discover and nurture the small voice deep within. This spiritual message center assures the contemplative person that a movement from self to other is life enhancing, so the "retreat" into contemplative activity usually leads to an increased need to be with and for other people.

The origin of the myth of retirement can be traced back at least to the Western world's first fixing of a retirement age at 65 years, which was set by Otto Von Bismarck, the first chancellor of the German Empire in the 19th Century. "Legend says that Bismarck picked that age as a way of removing political rivals older than himself." (Cohen, 2000, p.349). I believe that social security in its modern form was designed as a response to industrialization, which caused large numbers of people to become dependent for their security solely on earnings from employment. In the United States retirement was a concept created by the government when they created the Social Security system in 1935 at a time when people lived to be about 60 years old. It is not clear to me why people began to assume that once reaching retirement age and quitting work, they would be able to enjoy life more. We remain creative and vital people until death.

During that long period of life between our retirement date and the day we die, we are no less in need of feeling valuable, potent or significant than we did at age 30. Increasing longevity now dictates for most of us a four stage second half of life. First we take about three years in transition from our mid-life job to the next stage. We spend "fifteen years in active living, ten years in slowing down and two in assisted living. Active living...is the time to fulfill dreams and create new ones. These are days of excitement, achievement and risk taking" (Chapman, 1986, pp.6-7). The myth that has developed through history was that if we quit working at around age 60, we could avoid the drudgery of work, collect social security checks from the government and play, and do all the things we had been putting off and travel the rest of our life.

One problem is that in the West, we don't think of people in their 50's, 60's and 70's as being interested in self-development and spiritual growth. In China, men past the age of 50 are expected to seek self development and make spiritual worship their highest priority. "The older man is the center of contemplation, dwelling...on the action and the power of God" (Gutmann, p.91). "Aging" in the West includes the assumption that around age 50 we begin an inevitable depletion emotionally, physically, spiritually and intellectually.

When we age "successfully", however, we let loose the stereotype of retirement. "Successful aging" is an activity-oriented approach that increases physical vigor, that includes continued intellectual growth, that calms emotionally. Life-long, yet meaningful work and adequate recreation are also aspects of successful aging. "...successful aging means giving to others joyously whenever one is able, receiving from others gratefully whenever one needs it, and being greedy enough to develop one's own self in between" (Valliant, 2002, p.61). The problem we face with expanded life spans and increased health is that we have considerably more time to utilize our creative energy. We must keep working! This means that we need to shift our thinking from work as a job to work as satisfying ways of being creative, that is, good work. Those who age successfully have a psycho-spiritual model of living that enables them "to complete their life journey, harvest the wisdom of their years and transmit a legacy to future generations" (Schachter-Shalomi, p.5). Schachter-Shalomi says life completion, harvesting long life and leaving a legacy are three aspects of good work.

In Creation Spirituality there arises a tenet called "reinvention of work". The goal here is to consider both inner and outer work. "The inner work refers to that large world within our souls or selves; the outer is what we give birth to or interact with outside of ourselves" (Fox, 1994, p.20). Utilizing retirement as a paradigm for the Newest Age risks our believing that we are done working. In many ways, embracing the role of elder means our true work has just begun.

There are three ways to be an older person. Most are "older people". Some are elderly. Some tap the archetypal elder within and demonstrate proof of their growth into elderhood. The elder models the archetypal standard of celebrating life. They find doing good works to be more than a means to earn money—they discover a joyful expression of self in doing good work. They ring the bell for the manner in which one creates a cooperative community by living in harmony and making decisions using consensus. They respect Earth and adore the children. Elder expression has at least four callings: celebrant (sources of blessing) and mentor referred to earlier in this chapter and then wisdomkeeper and earthkeeper.

Wisdomkeeping

A wisdomkeeper knows that *w*isdom needs to be shared and that their story needs to be told. These expressions of elder energy are extensions of the spiritual journey. We are spiritual beings who choose a time on Earth to experience our human journey. As we center we rediscover our goodness and find that place inside that is connected, universal and ancient. The elder walk takes us closer to the center. Our connectedness and the peace we find at our center stir us to honor our surroundings including the land and the beings that walk the land.

An elder is at minimum a wisdomkeeper. The wisdom they store must be shared, but the wisdomkeeper only qualifies as an elder if the recipient of their wisdom is open to being influenced by their knowledge and insight. The elder in older societies was obligated by tradition to pass on her knowledge of the community's history. It mattered little how balanced the older people were when it came to passing on oral tradition: the telling of stories was only available in verbal form because the written word was not utilized for this purpose or didn't yet exist. Even a frustrated and angry older person could tell their version of community stories. The more balanced and heart-centered a person is, however, the greater is their desire to share because of their passion for the success of the young. This older person is a wisdomkeeper.

> When October winds do blow,
> Then a man his wheat must sow.
> Thus must act a man of worth
> Who has arrived at sixty years:
> He must sow in young folk's ears
> Wisdom all their hearts to fill,
> And give them charity if he will (Grant Kalendrier, 1926, p.351).

Picture the elder wisdomkeeper at a family gathering. The elder has asked the family to gather in one room. Once they are all settled, the wisdomkeeper announces that they have a tape recorder going and that they want each person to tell their favorite family story. Throughout the next hour, ten vignettes about the elder's family are recorded. The wisdomkeeper tells a story as well. Through this ritual, which the elder sponsors, the family's wisdomkeeper not only created a place to tell their version of family history, but also facilitated a family process that added considerably to the store of family history the elder supervises. The elder wisdomkeeper then offers to tell more stories at the Fourth of July picnic where the family traditionally gathers.

My mother-in-law, who is eighty-five years old, is writing the story of her life. She occasionally asks several of us to read it and offer her feedback. In this manner, she not only tunes up the content of her book, but also gives the family an excuse to discuss family history with her. She gave me the idea to contact my father and ask him to do the same. He "bah, humbugged" the idea but I convinced him to talk to a tape recorder. He still uses dial telephones, so I wasn't going to risk asking him to talk to a video recorder. I got one tape from him with just one side used. Driven by wisdomkeeper energy, I came back to him with a number of questions about the material on the tape that he could expand on in a second recording. By this method I got the reluctant patriarch to fill two tapes. In this manner, a person "saves" themselves for their children in the belief that some day their story will be found to be valuable by one's heirs.

If we look for opportunities to tell the family stories and encourage the maintenance of family history, we take ourselves into the mainstream of the family. The extended family has disintegrated and the nuclear family is splintering into single parent and blended families, further weakening the primary unit that binds the generations. The elder, if visible at the core of their extended family, can't repair broken families, but does model for the children "how to meet life's challenges with "spiritual wisdom, grace and courage" (Schachter-Shalomi, p.220). One function of the older people in a family should be the linking together of family history and the family's present reality. The wisdomkeepers of the 21st Century have a new look. They don't fit our stereotype of a wrinkled Native American sitting quietly and occasionally uttering words that overwhelm with their depth and appropriateness. Today the wisdomkeeper looks like a person, black, white, brown, red or yellow who has lived a long time and has a passion for seeing people connected. They do everything they can to be the glue that holds the disparate parts of the family and community together.

Earthkeeping

Erikson said that older people are natural conservationists. "Long memories and wider perspectives lend urgency to the maintenance of the natural world" (Erikson, p.334). Thoreau said, "We now no longer camp as for a night, but have settled down on earth and forgotten heaven" (Thoreau, p.40). We are here on Earth for now and the older we get the more this becomes clear. We knew it, as children but got busy and forgot.

As the demands of the workaday world become less we begin to smell the flora again, hear the sounds of nature and desire a slower pace that allows a renewed sense of oneness. The earthkeeping elder wants to sponsor a recovery from our separation from the land.

There are three primary bonds to my existence: to God, to family and to Earth. My work and my personal happiness are affected by my poor, but developing connections to the Universe and to the "ground". Grounding for me means having a connection to Earth. Grounding requires understanding and being aware of my physical body (Helliwell, 1999, p.126). The ground (of our ability to make sense of all things) is the world. The anchoring aspect of the world is the physical Earth and I believe our need for Earth is built into our being. Our myths teach us that "human beings are rooted to the land and will become disoriented, suffer and ultimately die if uprooted. A person is not simply the offspring of his or her parents. Each individual is primarily an incarnation of the land, a spirit being who belongs intimately and specifically to the local geography" (Suzuki, 1992, p.188). We are of the soil and the soil is of us.

Being aware of Earth beneath our feet grounds an earthkeeper. I first heard about the concept of grounding in 1970 when taking a workshop facilitated by Stanley Cohen, a specialist in bioenergetics. Determining how well grounded a person was gave Cohen diagnostic information about how neurotic a person was. Being grounded, Cohen taught, is the opposite of being hung up or "not having your feet on the ground". If your feet are on the ground that is body language for being in touch with reality. This means we are not operating under illusions. Literally everyone is on his or her feet. In an energetic sense, however, this is not always the case. If a person's energy does not flow well, up and down the body, their feeling contact with the ground is very limited. I use the term "energetic" to refer to something like yin and yang, two energies in a polar relationship to one another or like chi, the vital life force addressed in Chinese medicine. Also, I believe that energy is involved in all the processes of life—in moving, in feeling, in thinking and in linking with the Universe.

In bioenergetics grounding means getting a person down to solid ground. People have a mechanical contact with the ground. In bioenergetics the facilitator utilizes grounding exercises to develop vibrations in the client's legs. The vibratory phenomenon increases sensation and feeling in the legs and feet. "This experience gives some idea of what grounding is about and that it is possible to sense one's self more fully in contact with one's base of support" (Lowen, 1975, p.195). Grounding serves the same function for a person's energy system as it does for an electrical circuit. It provides a safety valve for the discharge of excess excitation. Bioenergetics facilitators like Cohen would treat clients by teaching balancing exercises that both build up a charge in their body that was energizing. The goal of the exercises was to connect the person with the ground.

In the field of psychology where bodywork of this type is done it is believed that "the more a person can feel his contact with the ground, the more he can hold his ground..." (Lowen, p.196). "When we are ungrounded, we don't trust that we can survive all that we encounter in our path" (Helliwell, p.126). Grounding me by gardening or just digging is my side of the synergistic circle people dance with Mother Earth. "While it is true that the various members of the natural community nourish each other, and that the death of one is the life of the other, this is not ultimately an enmity, it is an intimacy. The total balance in this process is preserved. If there is taking there is a giving. Without reciprocity the Earth could not survive" (Berry, 1992, p.244). While I am accomplishing the completion of the energetic circuit that is allowed by grounding, I am getting fed by the hidden circuitry, through which pass vital flows of energy and matter in the biosphere: that part of Earth's crust that supports life.

The concept of Mother Earth, or as the Greeks called her long ago, *Gaia*, has been increasingly meaningful for me as I age. As a result of the accumulation of evidence about the natural environment and the growth of the science of ecology, there has recently been speculation that the biosphere may be more than just the complete range of all living things within their natural habitat of soil, sea, and air. The Gaia hypothesis states that Earth's living matter, air, oceans, and land, form a complex system that can be seen as a single organism. We are not separate beings on Gaia: We are a mode of being of Gaia. How we think is how Gaia thinks, how an earthkeeper thinks.

In 2003 when I turned 63, I found some timberland in the area called "the Gorge" through which flows the mighty Columbia River. The area is aggressively protected from development and there are few plots of land available such as the one I found. When I first walked on the land I felt something important. First, I was out of my head while there. Just as when I am in the garden I built near my home, I am not thinking much while in the land. Secondly, I was overwhelmed by something magical. I am in touch with a power and a peace that is only available to me while touching ground. I often feel while working the land a kind of exhaustion. I feel something physical and then I follow the feeling to something emotional.

In the Judaic tradition is a concept called, The Tree Of Life. It goes something like this: In the void of space, first comes a spiritual impulse to create; then, a thought forms from the impulse; then, a feeling forms; then, it takes physical form. When I am on the land it feels like I am working back up this progression of creativity by beginning with the physical form of Earth, the rocks, the plants and bodies of water. Could this be a reversible process that begins with Earth and connects us to spiritual impulses in the Universe?

The way an earthkeeper's relationship to Earth affects their work and life has three parts. It begins for them with how Earth grounds them. This leads to the reminder that they are Earth, or at least actively involved synergistically with the world that feeds them, supports them and connects them. It is Earth that binds us together. The earthkeeper senses that to ignore Gaia "is to get away from what binds us all, namely the earth and up to what might set us off from others" (Fox, 1990, p.50)

When I reflect on connecting to the ground, the first chakra comes to mind here. The first chakra is the foundation to the seven-chakra system and it is located closer to the ground than the other six chakras. The chakra system comes from Hindu tradition. It is a model for personal development that runs through seven distinct stages. The chakras are aligned up through the body beginning with the first chakra located at the base of the spine. Growing up "through the chakras" suggests an ascension toward the Divine "by gradually mastering the seductive pull of the physical world" (Myss, 1996, p.68). Earth energizes me in my work and relationships…it feeds me as I feed it giving back my respect and honoring its abundance…it connects me to all life.

CHAPTER TWO

The Elder in History

*M**en and women reach mid-life today feeling that things have changed.* Many look about and see increasingly healthy 50 and 60 year olds who will probably live until they are 90 or 100 years old — possibly more. An increasing number of people are entering the second half of life not at all clear about how they want to spend their expanded time. At age 85 my father and my mother-in-law are vital despite some physical depletion. They are of the generation that arrived at mid-life with a sense that being a "senior citizen" was not the first stage of dying. Their generation was the first to experience a new longevity in the Newest Age. Their parents, on the other hand, had just a few years past the date they quit work to settle their affairs before death.

My grandparents did not live into the Newest Age like my father and I have. People had not experienced this new part of life until the last couple of generations. It is a generation — long stage of human development. Born during the Industrial Revolution, my paternal grandfather worked as a ship fitter in a manufacturing plant making warships for long hours that compromised his health. He not only worked until age 65, but for forty years worked a much longer work day than his predecessors who had been subsistence farmers. He was very tired when he reached age 60. He lacked energy for and had little interest in improving Earth, fighting poverty, being a mentor to his grandchildren or volunteering for community improvement projects. I have no memory of time spent walking with him, hearing his wisdom or even standing close by him. He offered a warm smile but was always distant. It felt to me that he was somewhat depleted and that he didn't have the ability to connect with young children.

The elders of history prior to the Industrial Era didn't usually disengage from life as much as older people today in North America. On the contrary, they often became the interpreters of the moral sector of society. The disengagement characterized by my grandfather was evidence of the impoverishment of men enclosed into the factories. By contrast, this generation—long Newest Age we are living in the 21st Century, has the potential to be "the first step in a total process of transition and reengagement, a process that reached its natural terminus in [an older] society but that is interrupted or aborted" in a society like we see in the West of the 21st Century. (Gutmann, p.26) This "new class of the old" is freer than all other developmental groups before them "to write in their own unique and original part, to lay out the new pattern of creative liberty…They will see that as they are the latest achievement of the life process…they may…cooperate with it by specific conscious development" (Heard, pp.164-165). My grandfather's generation disengaged, pulled away and hid out in their retirement. They lacked pride in their wisdom. Before today's new class of the old can live their long life in celebration, however, they must become like the elders of old.

Western culture does not have a bar mitzvah at retirement. The transition called "retirement" on our social clock is an artificial stage of development created in the West by governments who defined when they thought people were too old to work. There is no ritual to initiate a person into old age because life after 60 has not been seen as a vital time of development. There needs to be a new emphasis, a new direction for older people. We lack role models for the role of elder so how does this growing crowd of elder citizens become empowered? If people want to learn how to behave elder like in the second half of life, they need to find out what is needed from them. What is it that people and Earth need from elders? And further, they need to ask themselves, "What has my life experience given me from which I can now synthesize wisdom?" To address these questions, let's look back at what we know about elders in history.

Biblical Elders

One of the oldest sources is a book that contains a lot of allegory that most Christians and numerous others consider compelling as an historical work. The *Bible* in its many versions contains references to a class of older people who served as overseers, watchers or guardians. In the earliest days of the Christian Scriptures, beginning about 50 AD, a body of elders who were appointed by the apostles or their representatives influenced each Christian community. They were men who were celebrated because they could capture the interest, devotion and confidence of others. Women had not been honored in this way for a couple of millennia before which time it is believed cultures were "woman-centered, with the deity represented in female form" (Eisler, 1995, p.43). More on this below. Even the tribal chieftains were inclined to bend their will to that of the councils of male elders. This community structure copied one that dates back to the time of Moses.

The Mediterranean world at the time the Hebrew Scriptures were written was patriarchal, but communities in Moses' time were defined more by territorial ties than by family lines. In this tribe-oriented society, the patriarch had less authority than he had exercised in prior nomadic times. There was no king in Israel at that time. Communal decisions were the province of the elders, the heads of the families acting as a body. Moses had dictated further that to qualify as an elder one must be wise, shrewd and tested. The elders were the older men of the tribe. The words eldest and elderly, which come from the word elder, refer to older people, suggesting that the elders of the Bible were among the oldest. Given that the life span in 500 BC was half that of modern people, biblical elders attained the status of wise men while still raising young children, still new at their building vocational skills and still in the early stages of accumulating wisdom. Nevertheless, it was assumed that the elder stage of life for many was a time of making decisions relevant to the welfare of the community.

The role of the elder included hosting religious ceremonies, acting as arbitrators and answering questions about the proper way to raise children. "If a man has a stubborn and rebellious son who will not listen to the voice of his father or the voice of his mother... [they] shall take hold of him and bring him out to the elders of the town..." (Deut. 21:18-20). Moses' father-in-law advised him to draw upon the strength and sensitivity of these wise men "so making things easier for you and sharing the burden with you." (Exodus 18:22). Moses sought out the most trustworthy and incorruptible for the job. Age and prosperity were only two factors leading to the selection of an elder.

In the Christian Scriptures, the Apostle Paul wrote in the book of Timothy that to be an elder is noble work and required a man of impeccable character. The elder was considered nearly beyond reproach. For example, any accusation of wrongdoing by an elder had to be supported by at least two witnesses. Character was judged in part by the elder's commitment to having one wife and well-behaved children. Those selected were temperate, courteous, hospitable and even-tempered. Elders were to be "hospitable and a friend of all that is good, sensible, moral, devout and self-controlled..." (Titus 1:5-9). To become an elder, a man did not apparently need to be of high social class. The villages of the eastern Mediterranean in the first centuries after the birth of Christ were not highly stratified. Despite the fact that some older Israelites or Egyptians held property, stock and other measures of wealth, this was not a determinant for selection as an elder. The elder "must not be a lover of money." (I Timothy 3:4). "The love of money is the root of all evils..." (I Timothy 6:10). The most honored function of the elder was to teach.

The teaching done by an elder was to be spiritual in nature; their job was to interpret for the student the highest and purest moral nature of humans. The elder of biblical times was concerned with the sacred and was often believed to be God's representative. So our earliest model for the role of sage is a spiritual person. An older, more popular term would be holy man but this limits our view to spiritual people of the male gender. Also, a spiritual person is not necessarily one to whom we are necessarily ascribing a moral quality. The spiritual person is one "to whom the sacred is a spiritual reality" (Borg, 1994, p.32). The world's spiritual traditions all offer models of elders. In Zen Buddhism we find the *roshi*. Among the Russian Orthodox there was the *staretz,* who literally was a sage who functioned as a spiritual director. There was the *sheikh* in Islam and the lama in Tibetan Buddhism. In Judaism one finds the *rebbe*.

About 5000 years ago most honored elders were likely women. Until a few thousand years ago, when it was discovered that men participated in the conception of a child, clans of people determined their lineage through the mothers. The earliest religious symbols and carvings were of goddess like creatures. Men utilized their superior physical strength to protect the women who provided the men with companionship and shared in the tasks of survival. As time moved on and clans of people stopped wandering and began to collect possessions, the job of protector became more important. The role expanded to include protecting the family's "things" as well as the people in the family. The more things, the more important the protector became. Thus enters the pater familias, the male patriarch. His power was to remain nearly unquestioned as head of the family until the 18th Century. Some of these patriarchs were elders. Most were simply "in power" by reason of their gender and paternity.

In the Roman Empire, changes in family relationships emerged because of the wars that characterized the empire's history. The spoils of war had always been treated as the property of the soldier's family and were controlled by the patriarch of the family. With so many conquests, however, the soldier, with the increasing support of the government, was able to keep his booty and build up his own estate separate from that of his father's family. Additionally, women's engagement in decision making glimmered a bit as absent patriarchs were forced to share with women male responsibilities such as managing the farm. The early Christian prejudice toward women reinforced the power of the patriarch, however.

Women were often believed to be evil and unwholesome temptresses of men. St. Paul attempted to reinstate men as elders in the tradition of Moses in the first century AD. He taught that women were tainted with the original sin of Eve. In the 13th Century men, educated by the Catholic church to be physicians "began to compete with the traditional 'wisewomen'" who were accused of having magical powers that could affect health and heal (Eisler, 1987, p.140). Women were warned to confine themselves to housework and prayer. They were expected to unquestionably support the authority of the oldest male in the family. Even though in time women would begin to assert the equality of genders, for most of recorded history the male elder and the holy men have been the most dominant gender except for the spiritual woman's archetype known as crone.

The Crone

The three-goddess archetypes, Maiden, Mother and Crone, have been models available to us to utilize in viewing the life of elder women in ancient cultures. At three stages of life women have been the pre-pubescent Maiden, the fertile Mother and the wise Crone. Primitive people saw bleeding as a source of magic and power and this frightened them. Rituals abounded that facilitated a young girl's transition into womanhood at the first visible signs of menstruation. Her first pregnancy was also the transition into Motherhood. She was said to have held back the blood inside her to create life. The end of menstruation was a time of control of blood flow. The menopausal woman was believed to have retained her blood inside her not to make a baby but this time, to make wisdom. (Shinoda-Bolen, 2001, p.x) Since menses signifies woman's fertility, her menstrual blood is seen as holy, potent and magical. The retention in her body of magical blood gave older women in many societies increased power.

The older women, the Crones, became like goddesses and were concerned with healing, the dispensing of justice, divination, the care of the dying, preparation for death and regeneration. As patriarchal leadership reared its head in history, there was a demonstrated fear of the Crone. One of the early attempts to defuse the influence of older women was to confront extraordinary behaviors in these wise women as witchcraft. The archetype of Crone has, therefore, developed into an image of hag or witch and is not appealing to all women. "The Crone's title, Bringer of Death, also puts some of us off. That's because we're conditioned to think of death as end rather than a change of venue or atmosphere" (Morrison, 1999, p.11). Elders deepen their walk of partnership when they can accept that the physical body has a beginning and an end, knowing all the while that their spirit is eternal.

The challenge to our maturation presented by the Bringer of Death is an essential one as we will read more about below. Elders are more present focused. They "use the power of Now, which is the power of presence" (Tolle, 1999, p.136). This is possible in large part because of their acceptance of death. They might say, "Facing pain, allowing it to be, taking your attention into it, is to enter death consciously. When you have died this death, you realize that there is no death—and there is nothing to fear. Only the ego dies" (Tolle, p.136).

Clarissa Pinkola Estes celebrates the crone archetype as the source of women's intuitive nature. She says that because it is silent, has foresight and is felt by women in their bowels, it is called wise. This archetype is called the "woman who lives at the end of time" and the "woman who lives at the edge of the world." The energy of this archetype facilitates women's ability to be "both a friend and mother to all those who have a riddle to solve, all those out in the forest or the desert wandering and searching." This psychoanalyst believes the energy of this female nature emanates from the unconscious. This is the same region from which the energy of the elder within emanates. (Estes, 1992, p.9)

The Crone archetype arose within the collective conscious during the final years of the 20th Century in spiritual women's groups. For example, Feminist author Z. Budapest began doing initiation ceremonies for Maiden, Mother and Crone in 1976. In the early '80s, a group of women in Maine were holding Croning Ceremonies. Beginning in 1987, another group calling themselves "Crone," at one time 300-strong, banded together in Seattle.

Triads of goddesses were common in many pagan religions including the Greek Three Graces, the Scandinavian Three Fates and the Roman Triple Capitoline goddesses Juventas, Juno and Minerva—maiden, mother and crone. (Reif, 2003, p.x).

Magic and the Elder

In primitive societies, old people often enjoy an enviable position in the clan. They can possess an air of supernatural prestige. They, whose age brought them closer to the beyond, can be the best mediators between this world and the next. At the same time the beyond is also felt to be a domain of the forces of good and evil. Some old men and women in primitive societies were suspected of having evil associations and were even put to death because younger people feared their elders' netherworld cohorts. The supernatural prestige elders enjoy can have its dark side. People fear power gleaned from the unknown. This belief offers some insight about the ambivalence toward old people that is evident today in both primitive and industrialized cultures.

An elder's familiarity with sacred concepts and myth combined with the experience and knowledge gained from long life increased their importance in the ancient Old World, both East and West. In China, as an example, elderhood was believed to liberate people from the confinement of one's libidinal drives, set them free from the prison of collecting material possessions and promoted them to the rank of living spirit. Ancient elders often felt they should live unknown to avoid intimidating people and be respectful of younger people's belief in their supernatural connection.

While elders were often felt to have special power, the very old ones were also seen to be physically feeble. They were understood to have long life experience but would eventually become decrepit. "Impotent, useless, he is also intercessor, magician, priest, beneath or beyond the human condition, and often both at once...a sub-human and a superman" (de Beauvoir, p.96). Many primitive people feared old age just as much as 21st Century people do. Elders, who were the oldest citizens, reminded people of their own mortality. The ambivalence was apparent, for example, in the premodern society's prayer that their kings would live into old age.

There are many Babylonian and Egyptian invocations found in the *Bible* that move in this direction. Herodotus, the Greek historian, tells us of some tribes that worshiped their elders as gods. At one extreme were the Issedones who gilded the heads of their parents and offered sacrifices to them. At the other were the Sardinian people who disposed of their old people by throwing them off a high cliff and laughed as they hit the rocks below. (Fischer, p.6). Ancient people, therefore, had a mix of reactions to old people that left them ambivalent about aging in general. Elders were respected for their many years of life but feared both because they had special powers and they reminded people of the reality of death.

Oral Tradition

Elders have played a special role in maintaining a historical record of society. They carry a fund of valuable knowledge that is often confused with wisdom. The elder in cultures in existence before the written word transmitted knowledge they literally had to memorize. They educated the young by verbally passing on stories, myths and family memories. The elders presumed wisdom and experience constituted one of society's most venerable institutions. This is one of the most striking contrasts primitive cultures had with modern developed societies. The oral history passed on by the elders of early times was often very accurate despite the inclination elders had for occasional poetic license in interpretation. This excerpt from G.I Gurdjieff's *Meetings With Remarkable Men* gives us one example of impact oral history had on one boy who lived in the 19th Century. Gurdjieff relates this instance from his youth:

> One day I read in a certain magazine an article in which it was said that there had been found among the ruins of Babylon some tablets with inscriptions which scholars were certain were no less than four thousand years old. This magazine also printed the inscriptions and the deciphered text—it was the legend of the hero Gilgamesh. When I realized that here was that same legend which I had so often heard as a child from my father, and particularly when I read in the text the twenty-first song of the legend in almost the same form of exposition as in the songs and tales of my father, I experienced such an inner excitement that it was as if my whole future destiny depended on all this. And I was struck by the fact...that this legend had been handed down ...from generation to generation for thousands of years, and yet had reached our day almost unchanged. (Gurdjieff,1974,p.36)

Rapid social change and the process of modernization have rendered the oral tradition of many cultures obsolete. Much that elders know is no longer pertinent and much that they don't know is essential. For example, in Samoa the elderly are measurably becoming less useful as sources of information (Cowgill, 1986, p.173). Another researcher reports on the "'increasing irrelevancy' of the knowledge of elderly Mexicans" (Adams, 1972, P.119).

The old also enjoyed prestige because they were few in number in a slowly changing world where writing was rare. In an ancient elder's lifetime, their experience was never outdated. In ancient times people considered longevity a divine blessing. The Hebrew Scriptures is full of references that show the eminence and dignity of the elders. God told

Jeremiah, for example, to surround him with elders for they were wiser than were the priests (Jeremiah 19:1, 26:17).

Old But Not Always Wise

There is also evidence, however, that not all old people were considered eminent. "Great men are not always wise." (Job 32:6-9). "Speak, old men, it is proper that you should, but know what you are talking about, and do not interrupt the music." (Ecclesiasticus 32:3-5). "The wise man's knowledge will increase like a flood and his advice is like a living spring, [however], the heart of a fool is like a broken jar, it will not hold any knowledge" (Ecclesiasticus 21:13-17). Older people were few in number in ancient times when the lifespan averaged only about forty years. This increased the visibility of the elders, if not their preeminence. An archeologist who studied longevity by assessment of prehistoric skeletons found that 95% of humans died before turning 40 years of age. (Cook, 1972, p.595) No matter the life expectancy, there was always a group of people who were considered to be elders. The ancient cultures needed to believe in the power of the elder. Because the old in general were often subjects of religious devotion, "respect for old age [was a] widespread occurrence [in primitive societies]. Some degree of prestige...seems to have been practically universal" (Simmons, 1945, p.17).

There was also a stage of life beyond that of elder. Those who reached it were often treated with severity or, at minimum, with little respect. While most primitive people honored their elders, they showed little mercy toward the extreme old, the senile or decrepit. The people of Samoa, for example, buried their elders alive if they lived to this "stage beyond elderhood" (Fischer, p.10). Even the victim himself helped to organize the burial ceremony. In extreme old age people became useless in the eyes of the Jewish councils of elders because it was believed that extreme old age caused poor judgment. In eleven of seventeen tribes in Israel, suicide was a frequent practice in this last stage of life. (Fischer, p.10)

It was difficult in ancient civilizations to separate older people in general from the elders. It was the young who decided which of the older citizens deserved their respect. However, they were overwhelmed by traditions that honored old age no matter how limited an elder's apparent pool of wisdom. Romans asserted that old people were honored only on condition that they defended themselves, maintained their rights, were subservient to no person and to the last breath ruled over their own domain. Romans were not as concerned with elder wisdom as they were elder power. Seniority was honored even among the Greek gods, i.e... Age before wisdom. In the governments of Athens, Sparta and Rome, men spoke in order of age.

Far Eastern Elderhood

Early communities of peoples of all races were structured around the tribe as a big extended family. It was the foundation of society. The most honored members of the tribe were visible and present throughout their lives because the tribes were relatively small. Whether the elders were parents, grandparents or more distant relatives, their influence could be felt and their support sought whenever needed. Since the civilized world from about 1000 AD on was no longer nomadic, extended family stayed together. In the Far East, for example, Chinese family structure was representative of most of Asia's cultures. Up until communism became the driving force in the early 20th Century, the tsu, or clan "included all persons with a common surname tracing descent from a common ancestor. The tsu operated through a council of elders..." who usually implemented its will through the family's patriarch. (Leslie, 1989, p.87)

Unlike the Israelite elders appointed by Moses, the Chinese elder attained status most of all from the Confucian belief in ancestor worship. Older people were shown deference because they were the closest living contacts with the ancestors. It was believed that after death a man's higher soul, the Hun, became a mighty and beneficent deity. Participating in and drawing sustenance from the sacrifices offered in an ancestral temple by living descendants, the ancestor in turn guided and assisted his descendants. The fear that the Hun would not be able to continue a good afterlife, and thus become a miserable ghost without these signs of active worship, not only motivated traditional Chinese to make sacrifices but also to continue the male line. Males were the only gender allowed to make sacrifices in the temples.

The other compelling virtue that led to the honoring of older people in China was the Confucian concept of filial piety: reverence and respect for family. Filial piety was both a moral and social virtue. Children were not only encouraged to respect their parents, but also Chinese expected that they would in turn love their siblings. When they accomplished this, they would hopefully love and respect all humans, thus acting out of their humanity, their *jen*. Confucius said *jen* is what makes us human and forms the foundation for all human relationships. Reverence for the elderly in China has often reached the extreme, as this news story from the early 20th Century demonstrates:

> A Chinese man aided by his wife, flogged his elder mother. The imperial order not only commanded that the criminals should be put to death; it further directed that the head of the clan should be put to death, that the immediate neighbors each receive eighty blows and be sent into exile; that the granduncle and uncle, and the two elder brothers should be put to death; that the prefect and rulers should for a time be deprived of their rank; that on the face of the mother of the father offender four Chinese characters expressive of neglect of duty should be tattooed, and that she be exiled to a distant province; that the father of the female offender. A bachelor of arts, should not be allowed to take any higher literary degrees, and that he be flogged and exiled; that the son of the offenders should receive another name, and that the lands of the offenders for a time remain fallow (Dewey, 1913, pp.17-18).

Taoism in the Far East taught that old age was a virtue in itself. Taoism promised that aging took a man out of the confining shell of his own sensuality, to set him free from the material prison of his own possessions, and to promote him to the rank of a living spirit. (Fischer, p.17) In the Hindu world of today, a joint family system much like the *tsu* of China has survived centuries of East Indian history. The joint Hindu family is a cooperative at the head of which is the senior member of the family: usually male, but female if the patriarch had died. Often, the younger members of the family go to the family head and take dust from his or her feet as a token of the elder's blessing. However, both the family head and the family priest share the elder role in modern India. The Hindu family priest is a man who has studied in and graduated from a seminary. He is an elder citizen who is devoted to the traditions of Hinduism, the predominant faith in India. He is a living expression of the tradition of the four *ashramas*—the four 25 year stages of life.

In the third stage, the one occurring between ages 50 and 75 years, a person begins detaching from family ties, acquired wealth and societal roles. This is in preparation for the 75-100 year-old stage, the *sannyasa ashrama*. This final stage is most important to practicing priests who are devoted to service and self-realization. They are poor and supporting them is relatively simple for the family. The *sannyasin* eats little and desires little in the nature of clothing and other possessions. They are totally dependent on the support of others having given up ownership of nearly everything.

In India, China and other parts of the Far East the extended family remains the foundation of the community. However, even in these traditional cultures, a shift has taken place sometime in the past 2000 years that has caused the role of the elder to be split. In an upper middle class family in India, for example, there is a resident teacher and a priest sharing with the parents the responsibilities of educating the children. The teacher instructs the children both of the family and those of poorer families in the village. Therefore, the elder function of blessing is entrusted to the head of the family while the religious rituals are facilitated by the *sannyasin*. The education of the young is the responsibility of the resident teacher.

Parents in history have assumed at least these three responsibilities—blessing, spiritual guidance and education. The elders of Moses' time assisted families in carrying out the tasks necessary to meeting these three responsibilities. Mothers and fathers allowed the elders to assist because these people were believed to be balanced and spiritual. They were spiritual persons devoted to community first, and self, second. Even the *sannyasin*, who, in India, is admired as the ideal person who has renounced all worldly cares to attain the supreme goal of enlightenment, is self-selected. The elders of that time were honored and selected by the community. They were often shown extraordinary deference by the young.

In ancient Greece, it was decreed that a person was first a member of the community and an individual second. Socrates, however, put forth the philosophy that the need for the approval of and participation in society should give way to individual conscience. The aim of the wise person, he said, was no longer the plaudits of the masses, but self-sufficiency. To Socrates, "the wise man was not the one whose abilities had been expanded to fill his needs, but one whose needs had contracted to balance his abilities" (France, 1996, p.5). The route to self-sufficiency for him and his followers included a simplification of life much like that of the *sannyasin*.

Although Socrates is accepted more as a philosopher than a religious character, his principles had a significant impact on future spiritual persons all over the world. Socrates said, "I think that to want nothing is to resemble the gods and that to want as little as possible is to make the nearest approach to the gods, that the Divine nature is perfection and that to be nearest to the Divine nature is to be nearest to perfection" (France, p.6). Those influenced by Socrates believed that enlightenment or salvation required a denial of wealth and indulgence.

Indigenous History

Throughout the history of the great cultures of Europe, Asia and North America, numerous smaller pre-civilized societies have maintained elder traditions unlike those in more prominent cultures. The person who would accept the mantle of elderhood in the 21st Century can learn a great deal by studying the elders of indigenous cultures.

Indigenous people are the descendants of the original inhabitants of a given geographic territory. They generally possess a distinctive culture in which they have a profound sense of place and an active relationship with the natural world. While "modern" people struggle with allowing elders to have a voice, the oral tradition encourages indigenous people toward admiration of and dependence on the word of the elders. Primitive societies often still depend on oral history. They remain agricultural and not nomadic. Small extended families are the norm. In such places the elder is still accessible and moves at a pace more like that of the culture in which they live.

The elder in indigenous society has an opportunity to develop a deeper understanding of the interconnectedness of the Universe because of their connection to and dependence on the land. They assume that a force greater than themselves has caused the shared origin of all forms of life and the ecological integrity of natural systems. In his book, *Wisdom of the Elders*, biologist David Suzuki and his co-author, Peter Knudtson, expand the concept of eldering as an earth connected condition. Much of the next few pages is a paraphrase of key parts of their book. (Suzuki, 1992)

The authors found that indigenous people have a fearsome respect for the bonds of kinship between human beings and other living species. Domination of indigenous people by modern society over the past few centuries has caused us to devalue native thought. Primitive people's views toward nature, medicine, relationships and religion are unjustly maligned as being to simple or naïve, and irrelevant to modern people's needs.

The most colorful elder in both the ancient and present day indigenous cultures is the shaman. This traditional figure of spiritual authority is also known as the healer, medicine person or magician. This is not to say that others do not attain elder status. The shaman is like the senior elder who inherits the role of guardian of esoteric knowledge and is usually a technician of sacred power. The knowledge and belief system of indigenous people and their medicine men and women, has survived over thousands of years. It has worked for them and has needed little improvement to be useful even in today's indigenous cultures. The traditional behavior of the shaman is bizarre by Western standards and does not serve to make the native elder trusted by non-indigenous people.

In one primitive society known as the Caribs, for example, the young novice shaman must leave his home and go live with the old *peai* (i.e., shaman), who initiates him. The process of training and initiation can take ten years. The elder *peai* secludes him in a hut where he whips the novice regularly, making him dance until he faints. The novice is bled by ants and is driven frantic by being forced to drink tobacco juice. He then graduates after going on an extended fast. In both the initiation of a shaman and in his own healing, there is a pattern of a recurring series of trances, symbolic death, and voyages of his soul to other dimensions and, finally, an application of the knowledge acquired in the sacred world to a particular need such as healing or offering a blessing. (VanGennep, 1960, p.109)

Older women often played the magical role of healer in primitive societies. Among the Kwakiutl Indians of the Northwestern USA it is told that the sister of the chief became a shamaness when she separated from the tribe during menstruation. It is said that she met with her guardian spirit, Helemil, spent time with him in the woods and then reentered the tribe to act as shamaness. "She sang her sacred song, and then she bit four men and she said, 'I have been brought back to life by our friend Helemil, and he said to me that if anyone should make love to me inside of ten years, he would immediately kill him'" (Mahdi, 1987, p.232). After menopause in many older cultures women took on a different role because the community saw them as not capable of childbearing.

In a review of the processes we go through to select our elders, indigenous knowledge is relevant to our spiritually and our environmentally turbulent modern existence. Their magic may scare us or leave us dubious but it can work for modern people even though Western society and its scientists don't readily accept this. "We will always need the Native Mind's vibrant images of a living natural world that can penetrate to the deepest and most heartfelt…realms of human understanding" (Suzuki, p.230). Anthropologists believe, despite the cultural diversity of indigenous communities that, worldwide, they are bound together by a number of shared ecological and spiritual perspectives and themes, which form a kind of universal consciousness, a consciousness that brings forth an extraordinary wisdom. These include 1. Viewing nature as holy rather than simply temporal or wild, 2. Believing that spirit is not the expression of one Supreme Being but is dispersed throughout the Universe, 3. Assuming human beings are responsible for sustaining harmony in nature and with people, 4. Depending on natural cycles in time rather than progression caused by humans, 5. Accepting that the Universe possesses mysteries that will never be solved by humans, 6. Tending to celebrate the orderly design of nature rather than dissecting it for science sake (Suzuki, pp.16-18)

The indigenous person honors as their "most esteemed elders those individuals who have experienced a profound and compassionate reconciliation of outer and inner directed knowledge, rather than virtually anyone who has made material achievement or simply survived to chronological old age" (Suzuki, pp.16-18) Indigenous persons believe that older people have something to teach the young. However, they are clear that only a few have the knowledge of the orderly and harmonious whole that is the Universe. This knowledge, they believe, equips the mature and balanced elder to provide wise mentoring. The role of the indigenous elders Suzuki studied has traditionally been to facilitate rituals and provide support that assists people in becoming aware of themselves and their relationship to Earth.

In the Native American cultures of the USA the elders would be missed in numerous ways if they were shy about playing a role in the tribe and in their family. In the Seneca and Cherokee tribes grandparents are expected to participate in the continuous care of the children. In a traditional Cherokee childbirth ceremony still occurring even in the 21st Century, the "father and the medicine elders" conduct a ceremony "with him that served to bond him with the essence of his genetic father, the Great Spirit, the Grandfather Sun and the Grandmother Moon" (Lake, 1990, p.50). The baby is placed in a secure, specially designed Indian basket made by a "tribal elder who had gathered her materials with prayer" (Lake, p.50). The baby is literally strapped into the basket snugly with deliberate restriction to its arms and legs. The family follows a practice that is thousands of years old. They believe it provides the child with knowledge and experience it will need to survive. The baby is carried everywhere by the mother who consciously exposes him to her prayers, to his "uncles in a rowboat on the river while they fished with gill nets, and he has watched and listened to elders as they told creation stories and animal legends..." (Lake, p.50).

In native cultures, wisdom is found in those elders who experience life emotionally. For example those who have compassion for and are responsive to others experience life emotionally. The true indigenous elder is often capable of initiating intimate, insightful and understanding relationships with people. They connect with nature at the same time and don't find the two separate. However, the relationship between elderhood and old age has to be proven in the behavior of the indigenous elder. "Naturally older craftsmen have more experience in their trades... but...their knowledge [may have] precious little to do with wisdom. Of what use are instructions and moral sermons if one's capacity for feeling and compassion has been lost?" (Miller, 1990, p.158). Opening up to the feeling of being is a worthwhile goal for the aspiring elder.

In traditional cultures the function of the elder has not been limited to passing on concepts, but demonstrating the embodiment of knowledge. This awakens people and assists them in their intellectual and psychological growth simply because they are in the presence of a sage. The elder is there, they believe, to create conditions for an experience through which knowledge can be absorbed. Many modern men and women describe these primitive elders as irrational and intuitive because the spiritual elder's beliefs includes the position that a human's existence is a mystery and possesses dimensions that remains beyond human logic. Not only does the native elder believe that much of life's meaning is unexplainable, he or she believes that a human's make-up cannot be analyzed piecemeal. The totality of existence is not a series of individual parts that can be dissected for study, but a whole in which parts are integrated and dependent upon one another.

Those older persons in indigenous cultures who embodied the mystical beliefs of their community were often intuitive, perceptive and imaginative. Their perspective was holistic and believed to be boundless. Those who were seen as most in tune with these pantheistic and nature-centered mysteries were both feared and respected. This set them apart often and they were the model for our earliest ascetics like the Hindu sannyassin.

Spiritual persons of the first few centuries AD were enamored with both Hindu and Greek theories of renunciation. This in turn led to a belief in the maxim that harsh conditions of living were more natural and more conducive "to morality and happiness than the sheltered existence of civilized people" (Xenophon, 1910, p.32). There were a number of passionate spiritual people who appeared a few hundred years after the formation of the Christian church. Many were mystics who believed that extreme renunciation was the best way to salvation.

Hermits

A community of hermits began to form in Egypt and Syria around 400 AD. They have come to be called the Desert Fathers and Mothers. These people left their families to seek redemption and because of their religious passion and simple ways were often held by others to be prophets. They were not elders who had been selected by their people as in the case of Moses' people. They attained status because they risked their lives and renounced the trappings of contemporary people in their quest for enlightenment. It was believed by many that clerics who were hermits and who devoted themselves to years of reflection and the renunciation of worldly goods were more likely to learn deep spiritual truths.

Among the original Christians, especially the Russian Orthodox branch formed around 900 AD, the highest calling of the clergy was that of the hermit. In Russia the hermit-like clerics were called *staretz*.

By 1000 AD, the role of the elder had been redefined from father, mentor, teacher, minister and source of blessing to include hermit and ascetic. A devotee would have to go into the wilderness and seek out the hermit to take advantage of his or her wisdom. With the evolution of the professional clergy and in particular the solitary *sannyasin*, lama and desert priest or *staretz*, the concept of eldering shifted. Around the beginning of the second century, a change in family structure from extended kinship ties to a more nuclear family unit was evident in diverse cultures including Europe, Arabic Islam, sub-Saharan Africa, India, China and Japan. The growing community of professional clergy combined with a movement away from extended family resulted in a transition away from spiritual education in the home to mentoring by individuals who had made religious education an aspect of their professional expression.

Decline of the Elder

A contradiction formed around the clergy that began to compromise them and the credibility of spiritual mentors in general. "The vices of age were the vices of power—the greed and covetousness of economic power, the bullying and hectoring of political power…the arrogance of social power" (France, p.10). A person is tempted away from their spiritual center by exploitative power. The elder in the early Christian era had a taste of power because those who attained the status of elder were asked by the community to play a role in safeguarding and improving the prosperity of the tribe. The elders of numerous cultures formed into councils whose leaders offered an opinion on all serious tribal matters. The council was also often designated as a body of judges. In the Bible, elders are often described as being seated at the town gate acting as guarantors of the legal proceedings before them.

This evolution of the elder role is evident in the assembly of notables called, the Sanhedrin, in Jerusalem. This elder body of seventy-one men with legislative responsibility was made up of scribes and priests who gradually stepped in for the pater familias—the family's advocate for the sacred. The term elder acquired a different meaning in the first few centuries AD, because of the decline of the family patriarch's power from earlier times. In Greece, respect for the central male figure began to diminish as early as 600 BC. The young had gained greater legal and social independence. For example, Athenian laws requiring respect for ones parents were consciously weakened.

First Century Christian writers asserted that the authority of the *pater familias* was obliged to give way to divine authority. They taught that God was to be obeyed first, and parents second. The pagan families viewed the conversion of young people to the new religion formed to follow Jesus Christ as a rejection of family values. One of the Desert Fathers recorded this view on conversion: "But you say we must obey our parents. But whomsoever loves parents more than Christ loses his own soul" (St. Jerome, 1987, p.130). Another tradition affecting mutual understanding between children and their fathers was the high incidence of female death in childbirth. Increasingly the surviving husbands began marrying a second time and bore children by the second marriage. The age span between the father and his children was therefore greater in such marriages. So not only did conversion to Christianity erode the influence of the patriarch, age played a role as well. Many adult men had fathers whom they perceived as both old and frail.

The Challenge of Youth

The role of elder males was splintered and begged the challenge of younger men. It is the nature of males to be in a position where they are protecting others. Sometimes men compete for this position. Young men who hoped to share the patriarch's position of power began to deride the role of "elder". They asserted that attaining wisdom was not dependent on reaching a certain age and that many younger people were seen as wise. The elder's longevity began to increase his culpability because he was around long enough to commit many errors. Old age was beginning to represent a defect in and of itself.

Philosophers such as Diogenes and Aristotle were very critical of older citizens who had not grown into elderhood. Aristotle, at age 50, reported on prejudices in Greek culture that he found that were unfavorable towards the old. He wrote that Greek society looked upon its old as hesitant, suspicious, parsimonious, fearful, cowardly, selfish, pessimistic and avaricious. (Aristotle, 1959, p.3-6) Greek mythology often depicted older men as the enemy. The tradition of Uranus, castrated by his son Kronos, suggests that Kronos was justified in attacking his "elder" because Uranus' blood turned into evil giants when it flowed on the ground. Any old man with such evil in his bloodstream deserves confrontation and clearly there was little hope that he would grow into a generative elder.

The Olympian gods consisted of those who were either young or eternally in the prime of life. Homeric heroes were also young. Even the heroes who were older men such as Mentor, Odysseus' trusted friend, were honored because they were heroes and not because they were elderly. Homer's Aphrodite asserted that the gods hate old age. Both Greek tragedy and comedy scripts looked at the old as people who were in the way. The status of even the sages, therefore, must have been lower in ancient Greece than in the Hebraic world.

Greek mythology has few goddesses that embodied qualities associated with older women in particular. One exception was Hecate who is often referred to as the crone goddess. "She is a magician and a transformer, a facilitator, and a healer. She is a Crone who has come into her power" (Reif, 2003, p.132). The popular Olympian goddesses were mostly portrayed as younger maidens, not crones. However, in other traditions such as Judaism, Hinduism and Buddhism wisdom "is a woman, a crone and a feminine archetype" (Shinoda-Bolen, p.3).

Over time the potential of older people as a resource to the young gradually became underutilized. If the older person doesn't object to the prejudice toward older persons and does not utilize their long life experience to benefit others, they encourage the disrespect of the community toward aging and old people. In Greece more than in Israel, for example, history and myth tell us that older men attained high status if they participated in community affairs. If the old man was a judge, a priest, an arbitrator, a member of a council of elders or a teacher, the young Greek was more likely to hold him in high regard. This suggests that elderhood had evolved into a call that mandated service. It was clear that the Greeks differentiated carefully between "olders" and "elders", with the latter demonstrating their passion through active participation in serving others. The enmity of the young toward the old was especially understandable around 2000 BCE when the family patriarch had power. The patriarch had absolute rights over all members of the family, including his wife. He could, with the authority of a modern juvenile court judge, punish a runaway. He could sell his children as slaves or exclude them from the family. Newborn babies could be abandoned on his order. After having conducted an inquiry and seeking the opinion of other family members, the patriarch could have a relative put to death without any interference from the local government.

The Patriarch

By 100 AD or so, the Mediterranean world was reading the works of Plutarch, who integrated Roman values into his review of public affairs in the Greco-Roman world of the First Century. Plutarch recognized that the more the old monopolize power, the greater the impatience of the next generation. Throughout history the patriarch has provided an outlet for the accumulated resentment against old and oppressive fathers. The philosopher suggested, therefore, that elders not *seek* public office, but rather accept the appointment if offered. Plutarch foreshadowed Freud's concept of *"thanatos"*, the death instinct. The death instinct pushes older people to address their mortality and contemplate what tasks need to be completed before their long life experience ends. *Thanatos* energizes the elder like the *libido* energizes the young. In the second half of life, people are driven by both *thanatos* and *libido*.

Plutarch says old age's "most grievous fault is to render the soul stale in its memories of the other world and make it cling tenaciously to this one …and to warp and cramp it, since it retains in this strong attachment the shape imposed upon it by the body…Here old men especially go astray: once they have been drawn into admonishing others and rating unworthy habits and unwise acts, they magnify themselves as men who in the like circumstances have been prodigies of wisdom" (Minois, p.75). He was clear on one point in particular — old men ought not to retire from political life. Plutarch taught that older men were diminished in libidinal stimulation like sex and lacked lively taste buds. As compensation for this depletion in "life instinct", he assumed that compensation could come from the pleasure of performing noble acts. "It is a man's duty not to allow his reputation to become withered in old age like an athlete's garland, but by adding constantly something new and fresh to arouse the sense of gratitude for his previous actions, and make it better and lasting" (Minois, 1989, p.73). He was speaking about "new and fresh" kinds of service, not an accumulation of more political power.

Since in nearly all cultures the patriarch retained his power until death, it is not hard to imagine his offspring's' resentment building over time. Roman comedies attracted an audience of young men because these plays often satirized the struggle between the young and the patriarch. The impact on respect for elders was predictable. For the old it seemed that the more power they had, the more they were detested. In addition the greater their disenfranchisement, the more the young despised them.

However, in Rome a transition in patriarchal power began in the early part of the 4th Century AD. From about 320 AD on, by public law, a father could no longer condemn his children to death. In part this was connected to the increasing influence of the mother. Under Roman law, a woman could become her children's guardian where the patriarch was absent. Emancipation of adult children became possible as well. The father's moral authority remained high, but he had less and less legal right to control the lives of his family members. In that elders and patriarchs were often the same person in early history, the declining respect for the patriarch influenced attitudes toward elders as well.

In my opinion, four forces that led to the decline of the community's appreciation of the elder's influence were: 1. The development of writing and the decline of a need for oral history, 2. The formation of a body of professional clergy, 3. The institutionalization of education of children, and 4. Decreased respect for the male head of the family as women's influence began to return. As the teaching, blessing and nurturing elder roles were spread out among numerous players in increasingly more complex communities, our view of old people became more censorious. The parent's role as teacher and carrier of cultural history, for example, gave way to public mandatory education in the Industrial Era. The new respect for children, paradoxically, caused the community to create social welfare and educational systems that began to replace traditional family function.

Just because a man or woman had lived a long time didn't mean they had experienced life in depth. Most elders have used their long life experience to become more sophisticated and aware, while most of the elderly age without synthesizing wisdom from their experience. It became increasingly clear to younger generations which of the older people had depth, could nurture and could energize others with their passion for life.

Dark Ages

From the Fifth to the Tenth Centuries, historians found little to praise about humanity. This was the time when the Roman Empire crumbled and the Christian church created a powerful infrastructure more driven by fear of loosing power, I believe, than by a devotion to sacred blessing and the ways of spirituality. These were the Dark Ages, a time of war, robbery, famine and pestilence. This was an age in which elders may have been few in number. The leadership of both governments and the church were preoccupied with survival and exhibited few elder characteristics. Art was only expressed through the making of spears, belts and jewelry. Writing was minimal.

Notable exceptions to the paucity of elders who lived between 100 and 1000 A.D., however, were Hildegard of Bingen (1098-1179) and St. Augustine (354-430 AD). It was Augustine who popularized the idea of true old age being the time between age 60 and 120 years and that the purpose of old age was the renewal of a person's spirit. He was careful to point out, however, that living the Biblical life span of 120 years does not an elder make.

Abbess Hildegard of the Benedictine order was a mystic and visionary. A mystic is anyone who enters the mystery of life with wonder and awe that results in gratitude. One of her most elder qualities was to celebrate the light of spirit and offer a contrasting view to the dark predictions of the Church, which could not escape an indulgence with coming apocalyptic disaster. As an older woman Hildegard said, "Sometimes I behold within this light another light which I name 'the living light itself'. And when I look on it, every sadness and pain vanishes from memory, so that I am again as a simple maid and not an old woman" (Bowker, 1997, p.429). This passionate elder was also tired of being treated as a worthless old woman by the patriarchal institutions of both the Church and the aristocracy.

Wisdom in History

As people waned in their expression of service and focused mostly on survival, a hunger grew for elderhood's nurturing energy: wisdom. Wisdom is common sense in an uncommon degree. It is flair of insight and intuition synthesized not through fear and doubt but through love and hope. The Buddhist says that the route to accessing wisdom has as its stepping-stones contemplation, listening, reflection and meditation. These are also some of the tools of the balanced person living into the second half of life.

The mind needs to be quiet to access wisdom, thus the need for the stepping-stones of contemplation, listening, reflection and meditation. Elderhood is wisdom in action. It is said in the Creation Spirituality tradition that a prophet is a mystic in action. A person following a spiritual path who is lucky enough to be mentored by an older person is the recipient of elder wisdom. Wisdom is not something that is taught. "… for the seeker, wisdom is…indistinguishable from the pursuit of it" (Marcel, 1955, p.42). We are seeking, in elder expression, to "tap" our elder within and to synthesize from long life experience a common sense. Wisdom doesn't exist if it is not shared. The wise man or crone hungers to share their gifts. The wise person is interested in their relationship to their neighbor, their family, to those who know them and depend on them but also to strangers and to nature. They want to be accessible to all: both those who are moved by them and to those who are less enamored with them. They find themselves most alive when experiencing life among people with whom they can be a resource.

In Greek Sophia means "wisdom". For the writers of the Hebrew Scriptures Sophia represented "divine" wisdom, the wisdom of the Universe. The word Sophia is not mentioned in the Bible but interest in her reemerged in the mid-twentieth century when the Gnostic Christian gospels were discovered in Egypt. Sophia represented feminine energy. "Wisdom is bright", said King Solomon, "By those who love her she is readily seen…quick to anticipate those who desire her, she makes herself known to them." (Wisdom 6:12-14) When a male wisdomkeeper expressed this energy it was believed to emanate from his Anima, the female energy in the psyche of a man. However, Sophia may also be an expression of the balance of masculine and feminine energy in the psyche. The mystery of God is for me both masculine and feminine and transcends both. God creates "both male and female in the divine image and is the source of the perfections of both..." (Johnson, 1992, p.55).

The Taoist tradition from China contains one of the oldest expressions of wisdom, focusing on the balance of yin and yang. Just as every child ideally needs both father and mother energy in order to grow up in a balanced way, so every human being needs both the Divine Feminine (*yin*) and the Divine Masculine (*yang*) in order to mature. So wisdom, although felt by its first chroniclers to be feminine, is utilized by wise people only when it is expressed as a balance of masculine and feminine energy coming from the psyche and heated by holy spirit.

Wisdom as viewed by Buddhists is the expression of an enlightened person. A Buddhist who is on a spiritual path can seek to understand what is called Buddha nature. A Buddha is any person who has completely awakened from ignorance and has opened to their vast potential of wisdom. This opening and the realizations that accompany it is Buddha nature. Jews call this *Elohim*. Christians embrace the Christ nature. Hindus call it the self. Sufis call it the Hidden Essence. Wisdom in the East includes the "wisdom of all-encompassing space", the womb of compassion. Wisdom is mirror-like. The wise person reflects back to others an accurate version of what they spoke, thus allowing them to review what they said. Equalizing wisdom is the lack of bias. The wisdom of discernment makes it possible to distinguish clearly without confusing different phenomena. The type of wisdom that is only reachable at death, the Buddhists say, is called "all-accomplishing wisdom" (Rinpoche, p.153). These concepts about wisdom come largely from Eastern traditions. I find that Western men and women lack confidence that they have wisdom, period.

In the Christian monasteries that appeared in the Middle Ages, leaders were selected based on their merits but also on the wisdom of their teaching. Even at the risk of disdain for the older monks, seniority was often not a factor in the appointment of abbots. These professional Christians were not enamored of old age for its own sake. To them the "inner elder" has white hair. The inner elder was the energy they sought in their hunger for salvation and clarity about the meaning of life. Old age represented an abstract and symbolic problem of fallibility and depletion. The inner elder could be found in people of any age and represented both virtue and wisdom.

Christian philosophy in the Middle Ages included a spiritual purpose for aging. Although people of any age could tap inner elder energy, those persons over fifty or so were believed to have greater access to this energy. Aging was seen not simply as a process of moving from childhood to youth and maturity and then old age. Christian theologians acknowledged the possibility of transcending bodily age and reaching a more advanced spiritual age. Medieval theologians assumed that spiritual development followed along with the body's aging process. Anglo-Saxon literature of the time shows a preference for the wisdom of old age over the innocence of youth. The concept of spiritual stages of life allowed for a coexistence of physical decline and spiritual ascent.

In the Dark Ages the challenge of survival was great. It was not a time when even wise people could make much of a difference. Gabriel Marcel says the function of an elder is a "linking together...a bringing into harmony...The sage is truly linked with the universe" (Marcel, p.42). In medieval times, however, 1/3 of the population of Europe was killed by bubonic plague. In the wake of the plague, villages were abandoned, large amounts of land went untended and citizens revolted. The period from 1000 to 1500 AD was a time of constant war, rampages by bandits and mercenaries and the persecution of anyone who appeared unable to protect their means of survival. Large communities of people were discriminated against. It was such a desperate time that even generative elders could not be heard. It was not possible against such odds for them to link the community together and bring harmony!

What the sage seeks is authentic freedom. (Marcel, p.43) However, some creation-centered mystics such as Mechtild of Magdeburg reminded us that,

> The truly wise person
> kneels at the feet of all creatures
> and is not afraid to endure
> the mockery of others. (Fox, 1983a, p.69).

It was not until the end of the Dark Ages that people once again were able to define the role of the elder and the meaning of wisdom.

The Renaissance

Recovery from the devastation of plague, war, pillage and pestilence in the Dark Ages took place in the 16th Century. The process had an important effect on the credibility of the elder. The plague had focused its power on the young, thus leaving a disproportionate and larger number of older people in Europe. The survivors of the ravages of the Dark Ages regrouped to form extended families that provided protection for those left without family. This led to the emergence of a gerontocracy: a society governed by the old. The older citizen became a leader of families, then villages and then countries.

The older persons that might have aspired to elderhood were often tempted to enter public service in the 16th Century. An elder is devoted to the welfare of others and seeks opportunities to serve. Resistance and jealousy from the constituency usually accompanies a role in government, however. The more an elder accepted important community responsibilities, the more they were seen as obstacles, or rivals, to be feared. Older men in authority were often subjects of criticism about their diminished ability to enjoy worldly pleasures. Renaissance writers and artists commonly illustrated the life span with 12 scenes, each representing a month of the year. A man's potency and resiliency were shown to decrease beginning in the "fall" of his life. The month of August corresponded to age 48 when youth was seen as coming to an end. This was *harvest time*. At age 54, the end of September, the harvested grain is stored. It was believed that anyone entering the September of their life without financial means would be miserable and likely become a beggar. At age 60, the end of October, old age set in. At the end of November at age 66, a person shriveled up in preparation for death. And death was expected no later than age 72. Old people wise or not, were seen to be living through the tragic last stage of life.

In the 16th Century the Western world experienced a time of renewal in which youth was celebrated above all stages of life. Writers of fantasy began using the "fountain of youth" theme. Anything that suggested depletion or decline was feared. A unknown poet of the time wrote:

> Many are the miseries of an old man
> Who seeks a fortune and fears to use it,
> Who seeks the future and fears to lose it,

> Who lacks courage, spirit, fire.
> He is slow, inert, quarrelsome, querulous,
> He celebrates the days of his youth
> And condemns the youth of others (Fischer, p.16).

The Renaissance was a time of optimism and creativity, but aging ameliorated this period's fantasy of eternal life. Medicine, magic and witchcraft searched for utopias and wellsprings of youth that could stave off old age and death. It is surprising that most of Shakespeare's classic "seven ages of man" were stages that occur between mid-life and very old age:

> All the world's a stage, And all the men and women merely players
> They have their exits and their entrances
> And one man in his time plays many parts
> His acts being seven stages. At first the **infant**,
> ...And then the whinning **school-boy**
> And then the **lover**
> ...Then a **soldier**
> ...And then the **justice** ...full of wise saws and modern instances
> ...The sixth age shifts into the lean and slippered **pantaloon**
> ...Last scene of all...is **second childishness** and mere oblivion
> ...Sans teeth, sans eyes, sans taste, sans everything.
> (emphasis mine) (Shakespeare, 1928, p.360)

Unlike the elderly, elders are neither hungry for lost youth nor do they fear death. Elder like expression was, therefore, less visible in the people of the 16th Century than at any other time in recorded history. The irrational and fear-based drive to avoid or outwit mortality was out of synchronization with the advanced stage called elderhood. The model for the Renaissance man was the highly sought after condition called, the courtier. This young, courteous, witty, brave and assertive swashbuckler was quite a contrast to the wise, patient and contemplative sage or elder. Wisdom was believed to be a quality that belonged to the old yet old age was feared and jeered. The Renaissance was a time of revolt against medieval religious authority seen as gerontocratic.

The Renaissance was also the beginning of "modern history". Historian, H.G. Wells wrote that people in Europe began in this era to actualize a personal will encouraged in part by the widespread development of schools. Literature, news and other forms of knowledge were becoming accessible to the common person. Wells wrote: "The ideal community towards which we move is not a community of will simply; it is a community of knowledge and will, replacing a community of faith and obedience" most common during the Dark Ages (Wells, p.588). The elder of more ancient times could engender respect through the demonstrated use of intuition, sensitivity and patience. But, in the 16th Century and for centuries to come the elder in the Western world would also be expected to be educated and knowledgeable. To mentor or to act as a steward of life required that a person know about the nature of humanity. According to Wells, by the time of the Renaissance, people were informed beings.

The Church

The Reformation of the Catholic Church that was sparked by such men as Martin Luther brought a focus to the spiritual nature of elderhood. Good works were no longer believed to be a series of pious acts designed to secure salvation. Service to others and community was seen as a manifestation of an inner conviction about one's spirituality. In the medieval world, a person's eternal fate was determined by a priest's blessing, especially at the last moment of a person's life. John Donne declared in 1628, however, "our critical day is not the very day of our death but the whole course of our life" (Donne, 1952, p.58). The whole of a person's life became important. Martin Luther was highly critical of retirement from active life at any age. To him and his followers the purpose of existence was to utilize physical and intellectual strength to serve others throughout your life. He taught that this is what led to salvation.

Out of this era came a growing focus on the potential of the individual and less of a reliance on hierarchical authority and the priests of the church. The imitation of Christ like behavior led Christians to believe that an individual grows constantly toward the stature of God. This enhanced the view that spiritual growth is a continuous process of change or progression toward a more full life. Elders assume that this growth continues throughout your life. This Renaissance view of the world spread to the New World in the 17th Century. From this time forward, the history of elderhood was a Western world history taking in both North America and Europe.

Modern History

In Chapter Two we considered the impact of 18th and 19th Century industrialization on the family, on men and women and on older people. This was the time when the village and extended family began to break up. The impact of going to work in factories in urban areas of Europe and the USA changed the experience of families. The "enclosure" of people into the industrialized world was the "historical process by which a people are separated from their ancestral work and land..." (Kimbrell, p.30). Industrialization enclosed people into the cities and enclosed most women into the home resulting in an imbalance in the full expression of mature masculinity and femininity in Jungian terms. All of a person's "auxiliary resources were taken from him, and he was now a wage earner and nothing more. Enclosure had robbed him of the strip that he tilled, of the cow that he kept on the village pasture, of the fuel he picked up in the woods and the turf of the commons... They had lost their gardens ...In their work they had no sense of ownership ...The sense of sympathy and comradeship... the old village had been destroyed" (Hammond, 1912, p.10). With the movement of men and women away from the village came mobility for people in general. On the other hand the pre-industrial rural community contained few travelers. We would typically find families in villages of pre-industrial times and earlier having roots that went back for generations in the same geographic area.

Historical events have also served to divert our attention from our spirit center, our soul. In the 18th Century we were diverted by our interest in machines. The conversion was from a rural, extended family to a disembodied family with parents in the workplace and most mothers, who did not work for wages, enclosed in the home alone with the children. Our fascination with machines led to a passion for mass production and profit. Following the potential of the machine led us out of soul. Today men and machines are seen to be efficient, productive, autonomous, calculating, in control, tireless, rational and they act like they don't easily break down (Kimbrell, p.48). Making a living used to be a means to an end. Even though trading was an important aspect of survival in pre-modern times, selling goods with the goal of making a profit was not the means by which earlier cultures solved their economic problems. Economics prior to the 18th Century was based on exchange. Goods were simply produced for trade and consumption. About 1700, however, technology got more complicated. Thomas Newcomen patented the steam engine. Then in 1769, James Watt took Newcomen's idea and patented the locomotive engine. Off we went. It became easier to compete and the profit motive for the production of goods was activated.

Up until the 18th Century, agricultural life had settled into a system of tenant farming under large landowners. Side by side with the large estates, common land was used as pasture and for cultivation. With the approach of the Industrial Era in this century, the disruption of the traditional family and small community began. "For sustained contact with the 'world' touched men's innermost experience, indeed their very character. Many of the qualities most readily associated with success in work-ambition, cleverness, aggressive pursuit of the main chance-had no place in domestic life" (Demos, p.54). Ancient peoples were so connected to Earth, its flora and fauna that their innermost experience; their spirit was felt as one with God's creations. Thoreau lamented, "Who knows but if men constructed their dwellings with their own hands and provided food for themselves and families simply and honestly enough, the poetic faculty would be universally developed as birds universally sing when they are so engaged" (Thoreau, p.50).

Since the beginnings of civilization, manufacturing, construction and industrial activity had been the province of craftspeople that worked out of their homes. The specialists in the crafts formed into guilds in about the 12th Century and were their own employers, forming a large middle class. Whether they were farmers or crafts persons, the focus of men and women in this era was on creativity in the arts, trade and living from day to day. Capitalists, those who owned significant amounts of property and produced goods for profit, existed in small numbers. There were no rich manufacturers. The rich were the large landowners, moneylenders and merchants.

However, the coming of manufacturing brought a hunger for wealth because the power of machines made it easier to amass riches. People's interest in wealth began to take a toll on body and soul. Beginning in about 1900 men's life expectancy began to shorten in relation to women. Up until 1900 men and women could expect to live the same amount of time — about 50 years. The life style of men and women didn't differ greatly until the men formed into the great masses of workers in the factories.

The elder was accessible in the less mobile pre-industrial community. Grandparents, ministers, master craftsmen and older people in general could be sought out and accessed fairly easily by the young. The highly mobile 21st Century elder is often out of reach of the young. When I was giving a talk on eldering at a Unitarian Church in the year 2000 in Oregon City, Oregon, a young father said, "We would like to take advantage of the wisdom of elders, but they are leaving us in the dust of their RVs!" The rich source of wisdom called common sense has become more difficult to tap as families and communities began to spread out. Garbriel Marcel's once lamented, "There is and there can be no common sense where there is no common life or common notions, that is to say where there no longer exist any organic groups such as the family, the village and so on" (Marcel, 1955, pp.46-47). The interplay between elders and the young is considerable in settled, non-nomadic, relatively isolated rural communities. There was "folklore to be guarded and handed down, and there is religious thought, cosmic ceremony and rites de passage" facilitated by elders in small communities (Gutmann, p.217). This brings them honor and motivates them to serve.

As men changed their work focus from subsistence to wage earning and women were forced to take on more domestic duty to compensate for father absence, the elder's credibility shifted. The attitude of the young toward the old in general shifted away from veneration, to a greater sense of equality of people of different ages, and in time to the exaltation of youth. Our modern bias toward the ages of man is that the great challenges of growth occur before the age of 50. Western people have forgotten that personal growth is possible after mid-life and that long life lends itself to unique understandings. For example, "It is useful for us at any age to reflect on the purpose and meaning of our lives, but the summing-up phase of later adult life is uniquely empowering, because it embraces the complexity of decades of life experience" (Cohen,p.116). With a shift in our attitudes toward aging we usually find a shift in our attitudes toward the sage as well.

Indications of the shift toward gerontophobia, the fear of old age, include a sharp decline around 1800 in the use of grandparent's names for offspring. The abolition of meeting-hall seating preferences for the elder began about the same time. The first mandatory old age retirement laws were passed in the United States between 1777 and 1818. Laws structuring inheritance of property appeared in New England at the beginning of the 19th Century. In some respects the Revolutionary War in the United States (1776) and the French Revolution (1789) can be viewed as revolutions of the young directed at a gerontocracy.

The next great Western event that impacted elders was immigration. The older generation of Europeans and Asians were usually left behind in their native countries when the young emigrated to North America. Even those elders who did emigrate to the USA, Canada and South America were less able to mentor and model survival skills on the "frontier". Generational conflict was common among the immigrants who settled in North America because immigrant children adjusted to life in the new land more easily than did the adults. The young felt less attached to European traditions and picked up the languages of the new land more readily. Children began to complain about the elder's old country way of thinking. Whereas in Europe the elders modeled functional ways of thinking, in the new land they were seen as unskilled. Family heritage was not as meaningful to the young who wanted to become like the Americans or Canadians. The family heritage of the immigrants was largely rural. In America, however, immigrant families of the late 1800s were not only drawn to farmland but to the jobs in the urban areas. Cities, meanwhile, had been expanded, fueled by the growth of industrialization. Mills and factories were hiring thousands of unskilled workers.

The final great blow to the hearts of elder people in particular was World War I and World War II. On the fighting fronts the USA suffered 291,000 killed and 670,000 wounded. When I urge my father to talk about the events of his life, his greatest resistance shows when it comes to the years of WWII. He fought in the Pacific. He saw death. He can't think of a way to describe the abomination of war. It is evident that World War II had a permanent impact on his soul. Our fathers didn't feel good about themselves as soldiers because they were not archetypal warriors. They were extensions of war machines and killed with guns that are dishonorable weapons. To kill with the sword, the honorable warriors of earlier times had to confront their enemy, see him, and feel his heat. The warriors of WWII killed a distant enemy who was faceless. Many of their spirits died of the shame of mass murder.

At home in the West there were further losses. The rush to churn out planes and tanks contributed to work related accidents that killed nearly 300,000 workers in the USA and disabled one million more, many of whom were women and mothers. WWII reversed a trend of moving toward greater job safety that had gathered speed in the 1930's. As the soldiers lived in constant fear of death, homebound loved ones daily were facing occupational risks. These soldiers and their wives are, today, the last generation in the West that is living a long life with no sense of direction. More older people would have been generative elders had they not been wounded so much in the heart.

CHAPTER THREE

Elder Roles and Archetypes

*T*aking a break from a family gathering, two men walked slowly through the park. The younger man, Josh, said, "Ilene and I are going to get an apartment together."

The older man was startled at Josh's announcement. He took a deep breath and then offered a small smile.

Josh spoke again, saying, "We are going to try living as a couple before committing to marriage." He waited for a reaction from Dean, the older man, because he trusted and respected him.

Dean knew that Josh wanted a response. He finally spoke. "When I discovered I was in love with Linda, I wanted to marry her," thinking back on the day he realized he had fallen in love with his wife.

"It was less common for couples to live together before marriage in your day, wasn't it?" asked Josh.

"Yes," said Dean. "But, it wasn't convention that drew me to marry her. I couldn't resist. I needed to live with her forever."

Josh stopped walking, looked into his uncle's eyes and said, "I wish I were as sure about Ilene and me. How do you know when you are ready for commitment like yours?"

The older man reached out and touched the younger man's shoulder. He found he needed to take another deep breath. Many thoughts, memories and theories rushed through his mind. He felt the weight of Josh's question and wanted to be wise for him. He could offer so many opinions about love, commitment, and cohabitating versus marriage. His intuition told him, however, that his role was to be available for Josh, focused and supportive. This young man had placed Dean in the role of elder. He could escape the responsibility or give his all as a listener, wisdomkeeper and source of blessing. Dean thought that he might even ask Josh some questions that would help his nephew find his own answers. Dean felt called by the younger man, called to be present, gentle and encouraging. This is a call to elderhood.

Responding to energy from within his psyche and soul, from energy found in the collective unconscious which will be explored more below, Dean realized that asking a few good questions could lead a mentee to recognize the truth from within him. Socrates believed the answer created by the student came from within him "from a store of truth, which it [the student] already possesses unconsciously" (Taylor, p.149). Socrates also had considerable experience in mentoring. Dean was older and more experienced than Josh, but he wasn't sure he was being called upon to do much more than listen. He knew that the younger man would create his own answer once he was ready.

Women and men who express elder-like qualities have called upon their wisdom. This usually means they are more than knowledgeable but it means more. Elders have confidence in their intuition and are, therefore, able to discern what is most right or closest to true for the circumstance in that time and place. But even more important than demonstrating discernment, elders are sages whose sensitivity and maturity leads them to behave in such a way that those they influence are more likely to find their own solutions within.

When the elder takes the time to be present for a younger person, as did Dean, he does so in part to experience the quiescence of giving. Following this instinct requires that he be spiritually, emotionally and intellectually accessible which, in turn, requires that he be present. Being present means that the older person holds the container for the younger. Holding the container is a quiet, contemplative duty defined by psychoanalyst, Carl Jung. The older person who holds the container is expressing unconditional positive regard for the other on whom they focus and brings the energy of the Universe to the place where the two of them meet. The picture I get is of the elder holding a giant ball of light that surrounds the young person he or she holds dear. The light brings hope and an air of patience and support.

Just as the energy of the libido swings us into a tumult of activity expressed outwardly, *thanatos* energies of equal force press inward on older people toward quieting and soul-nourishing equilibrium. *Thanatos* is the other instinctual life force that drives us in the second half of life. It longs to return to a state of peace. These inward moving forces drive elders as they peacefully stand by while another grows or, at least experiences, a moment of confidence because of their advocacy. Martin Buber said it beautifully:

> The teacher helps his disciples find themselves, and in hours of desolation the disciples help their teacher find himself again. The teacher kindles the souls of his disciples and they surround him, his life with the flame he has kindled. The disciple asks, and by his manner of asking unconsciously evokes a reply, which his teacher's spirit would not have produced without the stimulus of the question (Buber, 1958, p.87).

Eldering, more than teaching, has the potential of providing the young access to a personal expression of self that links one to others and to the Universe. To teach is to impart knowledge or a skill in something. To elder is to nurture and celebrate the dreams of the one being served. Elders respect the knowledge that the young hold. The elder, unlike the elderly, thrives on facilitating the takeover by the young, passing on the legacy, for the young inherit Earth.

20th Century

As mentioned above, in the 19th Century industrialization of cultures began a massive change in men and women's roles. As people moved increasingly "off the farm" and into the city to become a cog in the new "machine era", they caused a shift in the structure of the nuclear family. Parents were moving away from the home during the work day, away from their children and often a void behind. The family home became more feminized as men's energy became less available. "Masculinity came to be defined less in terms of self-control and family obligation...

and more in terms of competition, ambition, assertiveness and virility" (Popenoe, 1996, p.111).

In the latter part of the 20th Century, women led us through a redefinition of women's roles that has impacted the Western world permanently. The paradox of this important change is that men have become unclear about mature expression as they continue to search for more balanced and sensitive personal expression. Warren Farrell writes in *The Myth of Male Power*, "Have we been misled by feminists? Yes. Is it feminist's fault? No. Why not? Men have not spoken up. Simply stated, women cannot hear what men do not say. Now men must take responsibility to say what they want—to turn a 'War in Which Only One Side Shows Up' into a 'Dialogue in Which Both Sexes Speak Up.' (Farrell, 1993, p.17). Male elders have also lost a sense of clarity of how to be.

During the 20th Century the potential arose for a new model of male and female behavior and interaction. Social change has escalated. In the 1960s, the sexual revolution, the peace movement, the civil rights movement and the women's movement among others occurred. In questioning old ways concerning our intimate relationships, patriarchy, imperialism, our treatment of minorities and the status of women, we introduced a more expansive human relations ethic that has redefined men's approach to women and visa versa. "Only then did self-esteem become accepted as essential to women's and men's health which was redefined to include psychological and spiritual health as well as physical health" (Myss, 1996, pp.185-186). Then, very suddenly, in the 70s people began looking inward for answers.

It was as if the high energy of the 60s broke down our barriers to introspection. Many people turned to psychotherapists, spiritual guides and other personal growth gurus. Then came the self-indulgent, narcissistic 80s. We rushed headlong toward finding wealth and speeded up our technological development to make life more comfortable, without thinking through the consequences. In the 90s, there was evolution in the air and hope that the next century would bring balance to men and women but also growing concerns about social injustice and ecological disaster. Creation centered spirituality became visible at this time. The Fall/redemption spirituality in Christianity had failed for many to celebrate the co-creative potential of man. Creation Spirituality tempted many at this time because it was concerned with social justice. I was less dualistic, less patriarchal and spoke of a God of delight rather than one who judges (Fox, 1983, p.11). In the 20th Century, we redefined gender roles, challenged the masculine and feminine mystique and brought more, but not equality to the genders.

21st Century

Still, we have not moved far enough. As the 21st Century has dawned, we must explore the possibilities for new expressions of masculinity and femininity that can lay groundwork for the future. Men and women must reach out to one another and take the risk that both genders can build a connection that honors gender equality and can infuse life back into the nuclear family and the extended family. Fathers must have hope that they will play an active role in raising their children. Mothers must have faith that they can trust their natural tendency to nurture and not be taken in by the call to wealth and power that rings so loudly in the industrialized modern world.

The family providers of the 21st Century have more complex skills than the hunter and gatherer of earlier times. Men used to be the primary source of the family's food and shelter. Today, men and women both provide. Today, we have institutions such as police, fire, and social welfare departments that are set up to protect our families. To teach our children we have created complex educational systems. Men and women have joined energies and talents to provide, protect and teach.

To speculate about what a 21st Century expression of elder might look like, let's consider a new look at the three parental role prescriptions to provide, protect and teach. It is important to remember to prepare for elderhood, men and women must seek to become balanced socially, psychologically, physically and spiritually. It is likely, therefore, that a people could accomplish this balancing in part by understanding and expressing in a modern way the roles of protector, provider and teacher. Consider these new versions of these three ancient roles:

Protector:
Being accessible to and supportive of your family and not separate from your spouse and children

Being Earth friendly rather than an exploiter of Earth

Standing up for ideals, beliefs or standards that will protect children and encourage them to care for themselves

Standing up for the equal rights of men and women

Perpetuating nonviolence and nondiscrimination

Endeavoring to make the relationship with the other parent of your children endure and grow

Provider:

Committing to share parenting and honoring the different skills of each parent

Seeking to find your passion and following it (This is the opposite of seeking wealth for its own sake)

Becoming aware of personal power (This is the opposite of seeking power in order to dominate)

Taking care of our personal health: physical and mental

Teacher:

Bringing to the family information about how to thrive in the world

Becoming a "spiritual elder" in the second half of life

Initiating children into adulthood

Sponsoring the process of integrating your children within the extended family and working towards building a family tradition of keeping the extended family connected

Negotiating roles in the family and at work (Assessing who in the marriage is best suited to work and who is best suited to care for the home and those at home)

Roles as Archetypes

The three roles above have evolved for centuries since the beginning of socialization among human beings. A model for human expression today can be found in archetypes. Carl Jung popularized the concept of pre-modern symbols having psychological meanings. He called these symbols, archetypes. He went further, however, to say the images created by the archetypes can be identified in people by patterns of behavior. People behave in predictable ways, he suggested, because imprints in the psyche govern the way we act. In other words, people are "hardwired" to express themselves in patterns of behavior we call masculine or feminine. The psyche is all of the human being that is not physical: the emotional, psychological and spiritual processes, conscious and unconscious, that make up the human personality. Our psychological processes originate in a community psyche called the collective unconscious.

The collective unconscious is a single consciousness made up of all our psyches connected by energy Jung felt was spiritual in nature. The worldwide memories and experiences of humans are accessible in the collective unconscious. The history of men and women is found there also. So the archetypes are common, repeated images that go all the way back in time and exist across all world cultures. Because of our genetic coding, physical characteristics reaching back to primitive life forms are inherited. Jung said this is also true for our universal, archetypal memory. It is inherited in the form of energies or behaviors. The collective unconscious is proof of God for me because God is the magic that connects me to others. I believe God is or God utilizes the ocean of the collective unconscious to make us all one now and throughout time.

Increasingly I speak about my spirituality in terms coined by Matthew Fox as he articulates creation-centered spirituality. "God is in everything and everything is in God" (Fox, 1983a, p.90) is a basic tenet of Creation Spirituality. In asserting this idea, Fox is embracing the idea of panentheism, a term devised by German philosopher Karl Krause in the 19th century to contrast with pantheism (Alcott, 2004). Pantheism recognizes the presence of God everywhere, but it does this at a cost. Panentheism says that all is *in* God; somewhat as if God were the ocean and we were fish. Creation Spirituality is both a spirit filled path and a movement, a movement that "awakens people and their slumbering moral outrage at the folly of our race" (Fox, 1991, p.16) and the damage we have done to Earth, to the plight of the poor and to the rights of the disenfranchised.

The pool of spirit that I dive into at my center is a bay on the edge of the ocean of creation. The collective unconscious is evidence of creation. The continuing activity we perform in concert with God is called co-creation. All people are connected through the unconscious ocean of energy I call spirit. The repeated pattern of behavior that is an archetype is possible because we act on what we know. In the process of tapping the energy of the ocean of creation called the collective unconscious, we act on what we know as products of history.

An example of an archetype is the elder. When Jungian analysts such as Dr. Allan Chinen discuss mature behavior, they refer to the "elder within". They refer to the energy within the psyche that influences elder like behavior. Chinen contrasts the popular archetype, Hero, with the elder. Our image of the Hero is someone who rides in and saves the victim or captures a great treasure. The elder, writes Chinen, unlike the Hero, "does not leave his or her dismal situation seeking better fortunes. Instead, fortune comes to him, in the middle of ordinary, everyday chores, and the elder's task is to be open to this unexpected magic" (Chinen, p.149). Here he is describing a common theme in old myths. It is in the stories passed down from our ancestors that we find ancient archetypes described. Jung studied myths, folklore and art in cultures all over the world. He found commonality. He based many of his theories on a study of comparative religion and an analysis of dreams, fantasies and pictures produced by people he counseled who came from all around the world.

Cultural anthropologists have catalogued a number of human traits common to all societies. All societies, for example, have laws about marriage. Ceremonies of initiation of young men and women are also found almost everywhere. Beliefs in the supernatural and soul concepts are universal. "If there is no human nature any social system is as good as any other, since there is no base line of human needs by which to judge them. If…everything is learned, then surely men can be taught to live in any kind of society" (Fox, 1975, p.122). While culture can amend the way we express archetypal energies, there is a basic, enduring human nature. Protector, provider and teacher are universal mature expressions that no human can ignore, but they have expressed differently at various times in history. There is a hunger that is hard wired into the psyche of people and it drives us to protect, provide and mentor or teach. To me the true nature of men and women speaks to us subtlety through stories, myths and even dreams.

When this phenomenon collectively regarded as the unconscious speaks to us from inside, it often appears as a god, a symbol, a monster or a vision of a man or woman. The unconscious, unlike consciousness, is a phenomenon of memory. It doesn't belong to the present. It is our history speaking in symbols.

For me there are some common archetypes representing elder. They include the grandfather, the crone, the sovereign, the wise man, the shaman, the priest and priestess. These archetypes have many of the Taoist concepts of *Yin* and *Yang*, the feminine and masculine principles which the Chinese believed permeated the psyches of both men and women. Yang is assertive and initiating. Yin is passive and containing. Yin gives form, like gestation, to the energy of Yang.

The female and male archetypes used most commonly have common qualities. The grandfather and crone can be crotchety but also parental, protective and nurturing. The Prince and Princess are childlike, innocent and loving. The Hero and Amazon are strong and assertive. The Wise Man and Crone are the mouthpieces of inner thought and wisdom. These archetypes are within each of us, are inborn and guide us through the our natural life-cycle—being mothered, being fathered, exploring the world around us, connecting to our peers, growing through adolescence, being initiated, establishing ourselves in society, dating, making a family, earning an income, participating in religious rituals, assuming the responsibilities of elderhood, and preparing for death.

Sovereign, Lover, Warrior, Magician

Although the Sovereign is the figure of authority and stands up for social order it has an aspect of elder expression. This archetype is also known in our stories and dreams as the King, Queen or Lord who directs and protects. The Sovereign relates to others as children or subjects, not individual persons. This archetype is a steward of life and is procreative whereas the Lover archetypes, Prince and Princess, are forever adolescent, with energy that is emotional and actively spiritual. These archetypes are seekers, preoccupied with his play and adventure. The Prince "goes his own way, seeks individual relationships and his own individuality, his own inner treasure, in ever new settings..." (Whitmont, 1969, p.182) More than Prince or Princess, the archetype of the Lover represents a complete picture of this childlike and, paradoxically, this sometimes clumsy aspect of self. "Our schizophrenic modern culture has a painfully ambivalent relationship to the Lover. We tend to accelerate a divorce from the Lover through a misdirected...spirituality, which takes us out of the realm of instinctual pleasure. On the other hand, we tend to approve of those who rush into the Lover's sacred space..." (Moore, 1993a, p.64).

Wise men and crones are often more concerned with knowledge and ideas rather than personalities or emotions. They are both examples of the Magician archetype. They can even manipulate and play with others to teach a lesson. They embody the intellect and its rational nature but also have an eccentric quality saying "social convention be damned". These archetypes, which are models of personal expression, can be found throughout literature. One of the best sources is in myths, movies and fairy tales.

Some good examples of the four archetypes are found throughout the three books of J.R.R. Tolkein's trilogy, *The Lord of the Rings*. Tolkien was one of our foremost writers of myth. In Tolkien's third book, *The Return of the King*, Gandalf, the author's version of the Wise Man, is in a discussion with Aragorn, a King:

In this excerpt, Gandalf counsels the King and encourages Aragorn to act like an archetypal King.

"...and Gandalf said: this is your realm and the heart of the greater realm that shall be...and it is your task to order its beginning, and preserve what may be preserved."

"I know it well, dear friend," said Aragorn, "but I would still have your counsel."

In the following excerpt, Aragorn is shown to be generative, a steward of Earth. He exudes vitality, which is a kingly energy.

"Then Aragorn laid his hand gently to the sapling and lo! It seemed to hold only lightly to the earth, and it was removed without hurt and Aragorn bear it back to the Citadel... And Aragorn planted the new tree in the court by the fountain and swiftly and gladly it began to grow" (Tolkein, 1965b, p.307).

The Wise Man archetype uses magic or what appears to be magic because of his powerful and unusual insight. In this excerpt, Gandalf is shown to be a magician who appears to have great power. His power, however, could be nothing more than illusion wise men can create with intuition and ken.

"He raised his staff. There was a roll of thunder. The sunlight was blotted out from the eastern windows; the whole hall became suddenly dark as night. The fire faded to sullen embers. Only Gandalf could be seen, standing white and tall before the blackened hearth" (Tolkein, 1965c, p.151).

Tolkein depicts the Lover in the person of the Hobbit, Sam Gamgee. In this excerpt Gandalf comes upon little Sam eavesdropping.

"How long have you been eavesdropping?" said Gandalf.

"Eavesdropping, sir? [said Sam] I don't follow you, begging your pardon. There ain't no eaves at Bag End, and that's a fact."

"Don't be a fool! What have you heard, and why did you listen?" Gandalf's eyes flashed.

"Mr. Frodo, sir!" cried Sam quaking. "Don't let him hurt me, sir! Don't let him turn me into anything unnatural! My old dad would take on so. I meant no harm, on my honour sir!"

Gandalf and Frodo continued to press Sam for a response.

"I listened because I couldn't help myself, if you know what I mean. Lord, bless me sir, but I do love tales of that sort. And I believe them too..." (Tolkien, 1965a, p.97).

Sam represents the childlike, playful self. He is passionate, impetuous and is not always in control of his need for excitement. The Lover archetype is emotional and can be irrational.

The Warrior is found in the character of Boromir. This knight is driven by a need to protect and defend.

Boromir says, "I was afraid for you, Frodo. If Aragorn is right and Orcs are near, then none of us should wander alone...Are you sure that you do not suffer needlessly?" he said. "I wish to help you. You need counsel...Will you not take mine?"

"I think I know already what counsel you would give, Boromir," said Frodo. "And it would seem like wisdom but for the warning of my heart."

Frodo is careful not to do all that Boromir suggests. He knows the knight is brave but he is dangerous as well. Boromir responds sharply to Frodo saying,

"Warning? Warning against what?"

"Against delay," said Frodo. "Against the way that seems easier."

Boromir responds, "We shall fall in battle valiantly.... True hearted men, they will not be corrupted." (Tolkein, 1965a, P.514).

Here, Boromir displays his sense of commitment to something outside of himself — to fall in battle if need be for the glory of his King. He is proud of his high level of military skill and physical strength.

To explore both cultural and archetypal elderhood, it will be beneficial to select archetypes that are as worldwide and historical as possible, and from there, integrate them into the 21st Century version of the three roles of provider, protector and teacher. To develop a new expression of gender roles functional in the 21st Century, I believe one must make two leaps of faith. First we need to accept that culture has a profound effect on the way we play our gender roles, and secondly to accept that the basic meaning of masculinity or femininity is hard-wired into our psyche and is affected very little by culture.

As I address the question, "What is an elder?" one answer is that the elder is a good example of how the archetypes of mature masculinity and femininity look when expressed from the heart of a person who has considerable life experience. If a man or woman experiences a balance of energy from each of the four archetypes of Sovereign, Lover, Warrior, Magician, I believe they are approaching an expression of maturity that is elder like. Understanding the archetypes gives the older person another blueprint for the fullest, most mature expression of what it means to express elderhood.

As we review the nature of these four archetypes it is important to integrate the role of our "dark side." The expression of each archetype has a light and a dark side. The dark side is called the shadow by Carl Jung. Becoming all that a person can be requires identifying and controlling the shadow. Certain aspects of the self must remain inactive and held in the unconscious. These dangerous aspects are our shadow. When the shadow is directing our actions we are dangerous to others and ourselves. A life run by the shadow is evident in behaviors like addiction and uncontrolled anger and the exploitation of other people and creation. It is the shadow that allows us to kill, justify our savage acts, to exploit Earth and model immaturity for the young. The balancing that is elder like is not only found among the four archetypes but also between the "bright" energy of our psyche and the "shadow" energy of our psyche. We express energy from the bright side of the four archetypes but also from the shadow side. The Queen, for example, can be a tyrant as well as a generative leader. But a woman who expresses Lover, Warrior and Magician energy as well harmonizes the energy of the Queen. This can act to quell the dark side of the sovereign's energy.

To complicate this just a bit further, there are archetypes of immaturity as well. There are archetypes for childhood as well as adulthood. So we add a third step in utilizing the archetypes to describe grown-up people. Moderated but also enriched by life's experiences, childhood archetypes give rise to adulthood archetypes in maturity. In the growth process the mature person doesn't lose their childlike qualities. The childhood archetypes don't disappear. "The mature man transcends the masculine powers of boyhood, building upon them rather than demolishing them" (Moore, 1990, p.15). An impoverishment of men and women can result from stunted growth. The patriarchal, angry, detached, abusive men, for example, are boys pretending to be men. The adult archetypes have the capacity to initiate, control and mediate the behavior of men and women.

One final comment about archetypes: they are not simply intellectual concepts. They have a feeling to them and are, therefore, hard to grasp intellectually. We can't explain archetypal energy any easier than we can explain how an emotion feels. We can experience it and we can describe the experience.

Sovereign

As we review the energy of the King and Queen archetypes, keep in mind we are considering a model for the expression of mature qualities that is based on instinctual traits "and their response to, as well as influence upon, those traits shaped by environment and culture" (Whitmont, p.178). In history, wise sovereigns included King David, Gandhi, Golda Meir and Winston Churchill. These real life models were not perfect but expressed good sovereign energy often enough to be remembered for leadership and as a defender of social order, both of which are energies of this archetype. The Sovereign is the archetypal leader and the voice of the people. Although I am describing a form of energy from the psyche when discussing archetypes, in order to simplify, I will refer to each as "it". It directs and protects, heals and invigorates. It celebrates life and is, therefore, generating life. It remains centered, bringing order to those around it; much like a straight spine facilitates good posture. It can be considered idealistic or even naïve in his or her confidence and joyful spirit.

Two functions of the Sovereign are essential to growth from childhood to adulthood: these are ordering and blessing. Within the arena of its influence are creation and organization. Ordering is placing things in a proper and reasonable sequence. With ordering and blessing comes a kind of spiritual creation. Mythologist Mircea Eliade wrote that a central force that radiated power symbolized creation in ancient times. Eliade called it the *axis mundi*. Pre-modern people found a center to their land where stood a tree or a mountain and often placed the throne of their king at this location (Eliade, 1959, p.63). The sovereign is the conduit for sacred energy into worldly energy. It is as if God's power must travel through one's being first through the head, down through the spine and through the heart into Earth. And the Sovereign archetype is a route for this sacred energy.

In the following pages I offer examples of the archetypes in movies. The examples of films below are quoted from my book, *The Elder Within*. They are, therefore, examples of films staring men. Forgive me women. I feel, however, that these archetypes apply equally well to men and women.

In the film, *First Knight*, King Arthur instructs Lancelot, who is to become an ideal warrior once knighted (Lowry, 1995). Arthur's words are those of an archetypal king:

"Now, I know the truth," says Arthur. "You care nothing for yourself…no wealth, no home, just the passionate spirit that drives you on. God uses people like you, Lancelot, because your heart is open."

The king energy in Arthur assures him that Lancelot is potentially an expression of God because his "heart is open." Arthur's view of the world, his kingdom and his subjects is reflected in this conversation with Lancelot:

"I believe that every life is precious, even the life of strangers. If you must die, die serving something greater than yourself."

Here, Arthur displays his celebration of life and then teaches Lancelot the meaning of commitment. He continues,

"Better still, live and serve."

"The roundtable!" says Lancelot.

"Yes, no head, no foot, everyone equal. Even the king," says Arthur.

Arthur experiences inner order and hungers to affirm others. He does not desire to have *power over* others. He is the caretaker of his subjects.

"Lancelot, just a thought. A man who fears nothing is a man who loves nothing. If you love nothing, what joy is there in your life?"

The king's most prominent emotional expression is joy — joy with life. The elder energy of this archetype is shown below in the list of elements of its Bright Energy components. For me, the shadow side of the Sovereign, the expression of immaturity, includes the aspects on the right:

Bright Energy	Shadow Energy
Leader	Tyrant
Protector	Exploiter
Transfuser of sacred energy	Withholder of blessing
Celebrant of life	Fears new life
Centered	Destabilizing
Generative	Destructive
Ordered	Controlling
Blesses others	Degrades others
Potent	Impotent
Fatherly	Patriarchal

Lover

In contrast to the parental energy of the Sovereign, Lover energy facilitates companionship and community. The Lover is the expression of personal concern regardless of the collective demands of the people of the kingdom. The lover "goes his own way, seeks individual relationships and his own individuality" (Whitmont, p.182) In myth the Lover is represented by Tolkien's Sam Gamgee and by Peter Pan...both eternal seekers. The Lover's orientation is to love in any form, and it lacks boundaries in the search. The expression of Lover energy is found in the Roman amor or, the Hindu tantra, the complete union of one body and soul with another. But, it is also found in agape, what the Bible calls "brotherly love".

The Lover is the energy of spirituality. With no boundary to its search for feeling, emotion and stimulus, in sex, food and other hungers, the Lover is our source of insight into the interconnectedness of all life. It cannot but be joined with all others. This is its spiritual message. The Lover is the archetype of play and of being in the world of sensuous pleasure and in one's body without shame. This is the archetype of eros, Freud's "life instinct" and the energy that fuels the life instinct, the libido. Plato said eros was the yearning of the soul for union with the divine.

Robin Williams, in the movie, *The Fisher King,* plays a childlike and adventurous fellow who is a good example of the Lover archetype (LaGravenese, 1991). Robin Williams plays the part of a teacher driven to apparent mental illness after the death of his wife. He depicts a man free of inhibition, without social graces, who can describe the source of his sensations. Williams is one of the most playful and fun-focused actors in Hollywood. But he is also a recovering drug addict. Addiction is one of the shadow sides of the Lover — it often doesn't resist the compulsive use of drugs. In his personal life, Williams struggles with his shadow as well. Once addicted, a person is always vulnerable to the abuse of drugs.

At one point in the film, Williams's character is in the park with his alcoholic friend, Jack, who is constantly caught off guard by Williams's child-like behavior. Williams says, "I'm cloud busting Jack. Ever tried it?" as he strips naked in a public place.

"You concentrate on the clouds, lay on your back and you break them apart with your mind," he continues. "You have to be nude, Jack. You have to build psychic energy."

"You can't do this. This is New York!" says Jack. "No one is allowed to be nude in a park in New York! It is too midwestern."

"Come on, Jack. It's wild. It is freeing," says Williams dancing about nude in the moonlight. "The air on your body. The nipples are hard. Your little guy dangling in the wind."

"Hey, hey. Come on," begs Jack.

But Williams's character insists on running about and rolling in the grass naked.

To gain access to the energy of this archetype, men and women must also experience the emotion of grief. The route to the Sovereign's energy is joy but to be in your Lover energy, one must let go and allow the welling up of emotion that is trapped by unresolved sorrow.

Some of the shadow side of this archetype is, once again, listed on the right side:

Bright Energy	Shadow Energy
Playful	Lacks enthusiasm
	Disrespect other people's boundaries
Spiritual	
Sensuous	
Connection through feeling	
Intuitive	
	Addicted

Poet Kahlil Gibran reminds us concerning the Lover and its shadow-side:

> When love beckons to you, follow him,
> Though his ways are hard and steep.
> And when his wings enfold you yield to him.
> Though the sword hidden among his
> Pinions may wound you.
> And when he speaks to you believe in him,
> Though his voice may shatter your
> Dreams as the north wind lays waste the garden.
> (Gibran, 1951, p.13)

Warrior

The Warrior's energy is outgoing, assertive and aggressive. When making choices like "fight or flight", its response is to attack or, at minimum, to stand its ground and defend the boundaries. Its reference is the collective values of the community, the state or country. The energy of the Warrior is devoted to maintaining high principles and it has a commitment to beliefs higher than itself. This archetype is a "go-getter". It fights, strives and accomplishes on behalf of the community, the state or the ruler he or she admires. The warrior is not interested in ruling or in being receptive or wise. It is concerned with focusing personal will and is proud of its prowess in this effort.

Examples of the Warrior in myth are Lancelot of the round table and Sekhmet, a mighty Ancient Egyptian goddess, whose name means "She who is Powerful". Real life warriors include Joan of Arc, the heroes of the Alamo, Gloria Steinem and the samurai defenders of the Shogun.

In myth we often run across a Hero. This archetype comes close to Warrior status but lacks maturity. The Hero is a stage of childhood development. The Hero likes to impress others, while the Warrior cares nothing for how it is regarded, but rather needs to reach his or her goal. What the Hero does is energize the child to enable him to break with the mother and father at the end of childhood and face the difficult task of growing up.

To be willing to self-annihilate in the accomplishment of a goal leaves the Warrior with an emotional distance from other people. The Warrior can't make its strategic decisions if it allows passion or emotion to cloud its thinking. In this way, it is somewhat like the intellectual Magician archetype. It is so detached in its strategy that it is able to accept its imminent death. The Warrior is energized by the knowledge that life is short. The Warrior is enthusiastic about strength, skill, power and accuracy. It employs spiritual, psychological and physical prowess to win. It is "cool" in that it only uses as much energy as is needed for the task. The Warrior's confidence and commitment brings about an unbreakable spirit of will. Skill and discipline combined with confidence causes others to have trust in its ability and it energizes others.

In the film, *The American President,* Michael Douglas portrays the chief executive of the USA (Reiner, 1995). In one scene, he must respond to an attack by Libya. A counterattack could quell the enemy, but it would also cause the death of many innocent Libyan citizens. He has just asked his advisors what else will be hit in Tripoli if the United States bombs its target.

"Nothing, unless we miss," answers a general.

"Are we going to miss?" asks the President.

"No, sir", the general says.

"And how many people are working in the building we are bombing?" the President inquires nervously.

"We've been all through this," a military advisor states in a frustrated voice.

"How many people are working in the damn building?" the President responds angrily.

"I have the numbers here, Mr. President," reports an associate.

"What shift has the fewest people, the night shift, right?" retorts the President.

"By far, sir," the associate says.

"What time does the night shift start?" asks the President.

"They are on right now, sir," responds the associate.

The President stares into space for a moment, takes a deep breath. A general says to him, "Mr. President?"

"Attack," responds the President.

The Warrior experiences emotion as a consequence of his decisions but those decisions are reached in a calculated and careful manner. The emotion that brings one into the Warrior's energy is anger. Anger doesn't characterize Warrior energy but one must "go into their anger" to find the Warrior in themselves.

The shadow side of the Warrior is contrasted with the bright side below:

Bright Energy	Shadow Energy
Assertive	Passive-aggressive
Committed to transpersonal goal	Selfish
Emotionally detached	Cruel
Strategist	Too concrete
Knows his limitations	Hates weakness
Establishes firm boundaries	Masochist
	Cowardly and sadistic

Magician

This Magician archetype is the master of knowledge. The Magician is idea-oriented rather than person-oriented. The Magician listens, receives, and perceives. It is a scholar, teacher, seer and philosopher. The Magician is the expression of a person's unconscious. There is something eerie about the Magician as if it has access to knowledge denied to most of us. This archetype is, therefore, felt to be magical or mystical. It can be a source of inspiration or of confusion. This archetype mediates the power of the psyche more than the other three masculine archetypes. In history, Socrates and Hildegard of Bingen are good examples of the Magician archetype, and in myth one finds magicians like Ben (Obi-Wan) Kenobi of *Star Wars* and Cinderella's fairy godmother. A Magician is one who seemingly has supernatural powers. Mystics, doctors, counselors and ministers seemingly have supernatural powers, or at least, their confidence in doing what others find baffling can give that impression.

Some believe that "in order to find our own individual centers, we need to be able to access the inner Magician" (Moore, 1993b, p.111). The Magician's wisdom and expertise guide us in our understanding of self. So, even though this archetype is really "in its head", we need its focus on the intellectual to grasp the meaning of life. In many cultures the Magician is the energy behind the ritual elder that facilitates initiation ceremonies such as marriage, the ordaining of priests and other rites of passage.

It is from the Magician archetype we are moved to thoughtfulness, reflection and insight. Whereas the Lover acts on intuition and feeling, the Magician reads the world like a mathematician, a scientist. It is unemotional. It watches life rather than lives it. Through this emotional separation the Magician protects us from the boundless love of the Lover, the sometimes-naive joy of the Sovereign and the anger of the Warrior.

In the first *Star Wars* film (Kurtz, 1977), Jedi knight and magician, Ben (Obi-Wan) Kenobi, advises Luke Skywalker on the role of the force in the life of a space age warrior:

"Remember Luke, a Jedi can feel the force flowing through him", says Ben.

"You mean it controls your actions?" asks Skywalker as he tries out his light saber.

"Partially, but it also obeys your commands," responds Ben.

Skywalker tries with frustration to utilize the force but can't quite grasp it. Ben offers him a helmet that blocks's Luke's vision.

"This time, let go your conscious self, and act on insight," the magician asserts with utter confidence in the force, the universal power Ben understands well.

"I can't even see. How am I supposed to fight?" asks Skywalker.

"Your eyes can deceive you. Don't trust them, Ben suggests. "Stretch out with your feelings."

To access Magician energy, a person must face their fear. The Magician taps the unknown, the unconscious and the mysteries of the Universe. These are sources of frightening power. The shadow of the Magician has been repressed for the sake of mature expression. Its two sides include:

Bright Energy	Shadow Energy
Master of knowledge	Too much in its head
Healer	Manipulator
Insight	Illusive
Protection from emotional irrationality	Stands too far back from real life
Scientist, mathematician	
Shaman	Calls forth the demonic Trickster

These four archetypes are a rich source of reference when asking, "Who is a grown-up person?" I began this section, however, with a discussion of the three role prescriptions: protector; provider; teacher. Further, our task is to integrate both the archetypes and the roles into life in the 21st Century. Finally, we can demonstrate that elders are models of maturity when they exhibit a balanced and modern expression of these archetypes and roles.

We can find the four archetypes in each of the three roles. The role of protector is a Sovereign in its stewardship of people and Earth. The protector is a Lover as it experiences passion for being with the family and strives to keep it together by working hand-in-hand with his spouse. It is a Warrior when standing up for ideals and standards that make his or her children safer as they grow and experience adulthood. It is a Magician when articulating the rights of women and children.

The provider is Sovereign like as she finds the source of her personal power and does not seek power for her own sake. It is Lover-like as it seeks its passion in life and follows it. Passion is far more important to the Lover in us than is wealth or things we accumulate. The provider utilizes Warrior energy as it cares for its health, both physical and psychological.

The Warrior knows it must be fit to tackle the job of living a long life. The provider utilizes Magician energy as it joins with its mate to assess who is best suited to care for the home with gender being a minor part of the equation.

The teacher role and the Magician archetype are very similar. In the traditional cultures of pre-modern times the men found themselves "on the perimeter" of the community protecting. Women have been found more often at the center in the roles of teacher and source of nurture. As the men were defending the village they also were assessing the nature of the world that lay beyond the edge of the community and then taught it to the young. A workingman or woman "out on the perimeter" today can bring home a description of the world beyond the home. This teacher can teach about law, politics, culture and earning a living. The teachers "at the center", in the home, teach about religion, morality and community.

The Masculine and the Feminine

Finally, as we seek a more 21st Century expression of maturity, we must address it as a process requiring the expression of the feminine and masculine energy in us and in interplay with people of both genders. One will recall that the feminine energy in men's psyche is called the anima. This is the unconscious feminine side of men. In women, the unconscious masculine energy comes from their animus. When a man experiences an attraction to a specific woman, it is often because she seems to embody his anima. The reverse is also true with women and the animus.

Over the past few generations, men and women have changed their expression both of gender and of energy. For example, women have made a shift toward birthing more often out of wedlock. The numbers are increasing annually. This requires that the single parent female to tap her animus more often if she wants to give her children a mixture of energy. To model for her children a passion for achievement, for example, she needs masculine energy. To model an appreciation for beauty in nature, on the other hand, she can spontaneously act on her femininity, for this is more natural to a woman than a man. A spontaneous, natural expression of masculinity is problem solving. It has benefited modern men in tackling the problem of harassment, for example. Men are increasingly addressing their inclination to harass females in the workplace. To be more loving, respectful and anxious to relate to women as equals rather than sexual objects, they have drawn upon their anima.

The people who will move about in the 21st Century with the most ease are those who accept the changes that have occurred in men and women in the last few decades honoring the archetypal feminine as much as the masculine. Relating to people of the other gender is another dual process: addressing both the person as gender and as someone who expresses archetypal feminine and masculine energies. Therefore, let's review what has been historically called masculine and feminine, keeping in mind these are behaviors that are not gender focused.

Masculine	Feminine
Values power, competency, Values efficiency and achievement	Values communicating, Values beauty and relationship
Is driving	Is nurturing
Is concrete	Is intuitive
Needs to leave it alone if it is working	Enjoys out-of-doors and sports
Is spirituality oriented	
Keeps problems to himself	Wants to talk it out
Views talking as competition, a negotiation of status and a preservation of one's independence	Views talking as relaxing
Hunter	Gatherer
Offers solutions	Wants to ventilate
Fears giving	Fears receiving
Is challenged by and conquers in the sexual arena	Sees sex as part of a love relationship
Communicates literally	Communicates figuratively

Some argue that certain behaviors remain more natural to one gender than another. No matter our focus remains free to move more to energies and less to gender. A 21st Century mature expression requires an adaptation to the changes in gender expression that were wrought by the social revolutions of the 1960s, the introspection of the 1970s, the self-indulgence of the 1980s and the millennial threshold of the 1990s.

A task of 21st Century elderhood is to integrate as much of the five processes discussed above into their self-expression. The five processes again are:

1. Expressing the energy of each archetype, Sovereign, Magician, Lover and Warrior in a balanced way against the other three
2. Keeping our shadow in check and not feeling too much guilt about having a dark side
3. Passing through adolescence and building upon the childhood archetypes to allow the expression of the mature archetypes
4. Playing the roles of protector, provider and teacher in a way that matches the needs of the 21st Century
5. Expressing both the masculine and feminine energies from with in ourselves

As we consider these ways of activating the deep maturity of the energy of the elder within, we may, paradoxically run into an increasing interest in our child within. As we sort out the sources of the spiritual, generative and wise expression that feeds elderhood, we find playful, spontaneous less politically correct behavior increases. Childhood archetypes like the Princess and Prince remain alive and accessible to us. In the search for more elder like expression we find that elder within and the child within are found close together in the center of our psyche.

CHAPTER FOUR

Elders As Revived Child

Elders are as old as yesterday
As young as today

As old as last night's rain
As young as the dawn of today

As old as their fear of death
As young as their hope and enthusiasm

As old as their memory of regret
As young as their belief in good

Elders are as old as their doubts
As young as their dreams

Bring old and young into one,
One in spirit, One with God.(Jones, 2005)

As we consider the elder, it is not so difficult to imagine the influence of the Sovereign and the Magician archetypes on elder behavior. The Sovereign is the conduit for sacred energy into the world. This energy from within our soul and psyche celebrates life and is, therefore, generating life in the way a wise elder does. The Magician is a source of healing energy, of magical influence and is a scholar, teacher, seer and philosopher. These qualities can make a good mentor. Less obvious, however, is the influence of the other elder archetypes, the Warrior and the Lover. The Lover, in particular, may feel childlike rather than elder like for it is sensuous, playful and impulsive. Paradoxically, however, elder expression is quite dependent on Lover energy. Recall that Shakespeare's final stage of development was the "Last scene of all. It is second childishness and mere oblivion" (Shakespeare, 1928, P.360). Maybe the playwright was hopeful that older people would loosen up and chase clouds once again. Maybe he simply wasn't biased. Maybe he didn't just think of aging as the creation of dependent and frail olders that bother others with their irritating and immature whining.

You will recall from Chapter Three this statement, "To complicate this just a bit further, there are archetypes of immaturity as well". There are archetypes for childhood as well as adulthood. So we add a third step in utilizing the archetypes to describe grown-up people. Moderated but also enriched by life's experiences, childhood archetypes give rise to adulthood archetypes in maturity. In the growth process maturing people don't lose their childish qualities. The childhood archetypes don't disappear. The mature person integrates the qualities of childhood, building upon them rather than demolishing them.

The Lover archetype is alive in us throughout all stages of life. The energies emanating from this aspect of self include playfulness, intuitiveness, spirituality, sensuousness, companionship and connection through feeling. Are these qualities any less possible in adults even though we often ascribe them to youth? The Lover archetype is more visible in healthy children than in adults but it is alive, never-the-less, in those who are elder like. What we see too often in the elderly is the dark side of the Lover: selfishness, restlessness, reduced enthusiasm, addictive behaviors, and disrespect for other people's boundaries. This is one reason why allowing elder expression to overcome our elderly tendencies is important. The experience of elder expression is more child like than being elderly.

Elders can be for the children a reminder of freedom and playfulness. One day I looked at my five year old granddaughter, Alyssa, sitting in her car seat in my truck, strapped in by a seat belt and required by "best practice" to sit in the back seat of the car. She was in restraint compared to how I was when riding in my folk's car in the 1940's. My children, Alyssa's parents, can't imagine letting a child be unstrapped inside of today's high-powered cars. It is becoming uncomfortable for parents to even want their very young children to wait at the bus stop without supervision. They can't imagine her waiting outside her school, playing with other children unsupervised until they pick her up. Is there a way that through remembering and celebrating our childhood freedoms that elders can be lighthearted for the sake of our grandchildren? Is it possible that an elder gift is modeling foolishness and playfulness that is at the same time safe? Is it possible that this is becoming more and more a needed role of older people as the young parents of today's nuclear family focus most of their energy on survival in a high stress world?

"Every adult...was once a child. He was once small. A sense of smallness forms a substratum in his mind, ineradicably. His triumphs will be measured against his smallness, his defeats will substantiate it" (Erikson, 1950, p.404). My youngest son Jeremy is now twenty-six years old. He is finding his way in the work world. He started a new job recently and within two days became anxious and felt insecure in the role even though he had good experience with the kind of work he was assigned. He said it troubled him that he would have fears like this, fears like those he had as a small boy. When he asked me about the feelings, I recalled the words above by Erik Erikson. While I wanted mostly to be a good listener, I also paraphrased those words for him. At that moment he and I both recalled the child within ourselves. We shared the reemergence of childhood memory and insecurity that never completely leaves any of us. In this way he and I were revived children, one and the same, son and father, elder and young man.

Children and elders hold the wisdom container for the community. My twelve-year-old grandson, Josh, was talking to me one day, making fun about his parents for my entertainment. He said that when his dad got angry with him he would say, "I warned you!" Josh, reported to me, "He hadn't warned me!" Often, Josh reported, his dad would step in when Josh's mother was attempting to direct Josh. If his dad felt that his wife was not maintaining control, he would say, "Shall I discipline him now?" Josh said, with tongue in cheek, that his mom would firmly and lovingly say to her husband, "No, I don't think so." This boy was aware of how challenging it was to be a parent. He was patient because he knew he was loved. He was patient because he was wise. At twelve, he was still able to see the games people play. In following his intuition he was holding the container for his family.

"The children, the young, must ask the questions that we would never think to ask, but enough trust must be re-established so that the elders will be permitted to work with them on the answers" (Mead, 1970, p.74). The elders bring long life experience. The children bring an uncomplicated sense of self. Together they can bring hope to the generations in between. The child is the promise of the future. The elder is the promise of long life endurance.

Elders and children are in touch with their spontaneous archetypal creative/imaginative impulses. Children don't become generative in the way elders do but, they express themselves more colorfully. Children are still young and still capable of knowing the world as wonder. "To reconnect to wonder is to awaken the child inside…" (Fox, 2002, p.179) and in this way the elder revives her child within and, like the child, models imaginative behavior.

Elders have time for a generative expression toward human beings and Earth because most of us are out of the work world. An aspect of retirement that older people enjoy is the emphasis on rest and play. Thoreau said that the "mass of men lead lives of quiet desperation… unconscious despair is concealed even under what are called the games and amusements of mankind. There is no play in them, for this comes after work" (Thoreau, p.7). Like today there was a dearth of elders in Thoreau's time who remembered childhood's play. The concept of "retirement" is problematic if we see it as a time of retreat that leads us to move out of the community and our sphere of influence. If we could retire with emotional and geographical accessibility, we might have a greater influence on the young children. Retired people are free to be more playful, less restricted by social convention, more spontaneous in their activities, more careless with money and should certainly be much less concerned with spilt milk. Elder expression is more possible, therefore, when we are free of the routine and energy output necessary in the workaday world. It is as if in retirement that the child inside us is returning to influence.

Child/Elder Male Archetypes

In the world of Jungian psychology a model for personal expression called the Puer is the archetype for eternal youth. Its opposite is the Senex, the wise old man. The spirit of Puer is uplifting, soaring into realms of divine inspiration and optimism, is full of visions, idealism and creativity (Preece, 2003). The Puer also is searching for a safe place of support where he will find support for his aspirations. The "old person", the Senex, becomes that place, becomes the structure where the Puer's visions and ideas crystallize and solidify into form. Senex is the archetype of practical structures and systems. Puer and Senex don't live easily along side one another and yet to experience life fully, they need each other. Elder expression could be a fuller integration of these two archetypes.

A breakdown of the coexistence between the two can lead to one or the other bringing about problems. The Puer can become self-indulgent, possessed with an immeasurable death wish, challenging the gods as demonstrated by James Dean and other icons of pop culture who lived dangerously. The old can get cut off from their "other" and adopt a rigid cynical attitude towards life. Peter Pan is youth. Captain Hook is old age. The lost Puer in Peter Pan led to the decision to never grow up and the lost old man in Hook led him in a vain attempt to escape the crocodile.

Peter and Hook avoid recognizing each other as the compliment that is needed to complete the ambivalent Puer-Senex expression. Hook, a bitter old man, is consumed by the crocodile and is swallowed by death before his time. Peter is forever excluded from consciousness, never able to gain an awareness of himself, never able to grow up (Miller, 2001). "Without the enthusiasm and eros of the son, authority loses its idealism" (Hillman, 1987, p.29). In contrast, however, the Senex archetype, in touch with the child within, offers wisdom. The Puer, if balanced by the opposite energy of the wise one, is playful, loving and the source of spiritual connection.

Carl Jung said that childhood was that state in which we can be a problem for others in our carefree and dependent nature and that in old age, "we descend again into that condition where…we once more become something of a problem for others" (Jung, 1971, p.22). We can let loose! We can wear purple! We can stumble and giggle with less price to pay in terms of social acceptance. This is an opportunity to be with the young, is it not?

It Is Scary To Be A Child Today

When I was six year old there was no graphic violence in movies and we had no television. Radio was unable to broadcast much that was very scary or intimidating. Media did not have a large influence on me. I was free to create childhood ideas and fantasies without the influence of loud, vivid, violent and penetrating media. Can I recall that safe and what some would call, naïve era and bring it in some useful way to the young? Old age "gives back an extended range of hitherto closeted pleasures, those of the table and the community of *companions...*" (Guttman, p.102). As I age, some "hitherto closeted pleasures" are calling me and making me more aware once again of joy and playfulness I knew as a child. But I was safer then. Today's child is born into a world where DVD movies of all ranges of exposure, in many ways violent, are within reach in the home. Children don't stay outside and play until it is dark anymore.

Chemical abuse looms and parents are called to protect the children from this menace. "Healthy parents are the anti-drug!" I see fear in the eyes of my adult children as they muse openly about the new reality we call, terrorism. This fear is not something they can keep from their children, our grandchildren. If we want to fear something, we should fear a loss of sense of child like awe. If we aspire to elderhood we must keep in perspective the vast differences between life today and life then while at the same time being aware of the qualities we have in common with children. Recalling our childhood makes it more possible for us to understand children and to avoid being irritated by their impetuous and spontaneous ways.

Recalling Childhood

Candy cigarettes were a big item when I was five years old. Today, however, we are concerned with increasing childhood obesity. I enjoyed sucking the sugary juice from Coke shaped wax bottles and was able to buy penny candy. Soda pop machines dispensed glass bottles and we had soda fountains with tableside juke boxes. My favorite drink was a Green River soda. We couldn't buy anything "fast". We not only didn't have fast food restaurants, most places were closed after dark and on Sundays. Eating Kool-Aid powder with sugar right from the pack was a big treat.

Elders As Revived Child

Today, however, Kool-Aid is just a bad example of a drink that has no food value.

Let's list some other assumptions today's older people make about being in the world when they were children. This is one way to recall our childhood, to connect with our child within and increase our appreciation of the children around us. When we were kids:

- Home milk delivery came in glass bottles, with the cream at the top and they had cardboard stoppers.
- Dial telephones had party lines, no area codes and we had a ring that was different than the other parties on our line (but we could listen in to their conversations if we wanted).
- Newsreels and cartoons preceded the hour long feature films at the cinema.
- Boys had a peashooter, sling shot and baseball cards that came with bubble gum.
- Girls had a roller skate key, jump rope and a Raggedy Ann doll.
- Television became visible in many homes around 1950 and the characters who we embraced included Howdy Doody, Beanie and Cecil.
- Radio was still big also and we listened to Let's Pretend on Saturday morning.
- In the evening were the Shadow and the Green Hornet shows.
- Toys popular then included Tinker Toys, Erector sets, Lincoln Logs and Hula Hoops.
- Parents complained about $.35 gasoline and trying to get regular deliveries from the ice man who walked right into the house and put the ice in our ice box.
- Children waited on the porch for the Good Humor man and expected only three flavors of ice cream: Chocolate, Strawberry and Vanilla.
- Children's games included Red Light-Green Light, hopscotch, Jacks, dodge ball, Mother May I? Red Rover and Oly-Oly-Oxen Free.
- Children made decisions by going, "eeny-meeney-miney-mo".
- The things we caught in canning jars were usually bees, lightning bugs and grasshoppers.

ELDER

- Around the corner seemed far away and going "downtown" was a big adventure.
- Playing Cowboys and Indians had no undertone of discrimination or prejudice.
- We played outside until dark in the summer and no one knew where we were most of the time.
- We had access to two kinds of sneakers: Keds and PF Flyers.
- We cut down our own Christmas tree just across town alongside the road.
- Nearly everyone's Mom was at home when the kids got there.

  It was a time,
  - When the Tooth Fairy left a dime,
  - When you'd reach into a muddy gutter for a penny,
  - When girls neither dated nor kissed until late high school,
  - When all the male teachers had neckties,
  - When we sat in the car while the men cleaned the windshield, checked the oil and pumped the gas'
  - When trading in Green Stamps was a true bonus,
  - When being sent to the principle's office was nothing compared to the fate that awaited us at home,
  - When it was magic when Dad removed and reseated his thumb,
  - When having a weapon in school meant being caught with a sling shot,
  - When scrapes and bruises were kissed and made better and
  - When the worst embarrassment was not being picked for the team.

Adultism

Elderhood is intergenerational. One could say that elders are selected by the young. They decide whether we are really accessible, passionate, safe and wise. The population in the West, however, is becoming mostly adult. The proportion of children to adults is diminishing. With increasing long life and a bias toward small families, adults have an increasing responsibility to children, therefore, to remember what it is like to be a child. The condition called adultism must be responded to in the way we responded a few decades ago to sexism and racism: as fear based assumptions that block our ability to connect to others.

Adultism refers to behaviors and attitudes based on the assumption that adults are better than young people, and entitled to act upon young people without their agreement. This mistreatment is reinforced by social institutions; laws, customs, and attitudes. Those who are victims of adultism were not challenged in childhood by a trusted elder to form a dream, a vision into which they could channel their talents and personal gifts. The increasing ratio of older people to children is a call to those of us who are aging to consider one of our roles in the Newest Age: to hold the dreams of the young when there is no one else available. Adultism is found in old geezers who are irritated by children.

It may not seem that long ago since you were a child looking at people who were the age that you are now and saw varicose veins, a bald head, wrinkles and dentures. Here you are, however, as old as you feared you might become. In the little book, *Geezerhood,* from which the following few sentences were paraphrased, we are encouraged, tongue in cheek, hearing things like "Yet you are not completely dead" (Allred, 1996, p.3). The amazing thing is, now that we are getting up there in years, we realize that being older might not be so bad. In fact, we look back and say, "I don't want to be 20 again...unless I get to take my experience with me." We could do without the loss of short term memory, back aches, bleeding gums, fatigue, weight gain, hemorrhoids, chronic indigestion and arthritis. Plus the financial problems can be frustrating. No one wants us working for them even if we still like working "which you don't because you're old, decrepit and beat up."

"If you're starting to 'geeze' you have probably concluded that, life probably could be a whole lot worse. At least the parts that you can remember...compared to the alternative." Children need us to laugh with them and it is easier if we can make fun of our geezerhood. We have diminished capacity, energy and disposition to deal with new things. Children can help. Just watch them. They have reflexes, strength, energy and memory. They contemplate the unknown without fear. "...the child thinks the sun follows him, that things are always as he actually sees them and independent of perspective...he believes himself the center of the world" (Piaget, 1967, p.127).

Children are present focused. The past is gone and the future has no name. They have the power of now.

An aspect of maturity that is paradoxical for the elder is the extent to which mature people embrace their immaturity. Older people once again become something of a problem for others as they were as children. Older people can't live in the evening of their life the way they did in life's morning but the child within is still alive. But, we need to grow up! The paradox felt by the elder is that "maturity needs guidance as well as encouragement from what has been produced and must be taken care of" (Erikson, 1950, pp.266-267). A child like nature is an elder quality but maturity can be defined as a state of knowing that comes from long life experience and where the older person seeks the support and the knowledge of youth. Within us is the energy of both our historical child and our future elder. The mature person experiences an awareness of a dance where, hand in hand, our inner child and the elder within move together in play, in grief and carry one another through life.

In his review of medieval philosophers, including Origen and St. Ambrose, writer George Minois quotes them concerning elderhood: "In Scripture, the name of elder…is…granted in order to honour maturity of judgement and gravity of life…Thus even in childhood there is a sort of venerable old age of behavior, and in old age a child-like innocence, because there is a form of old age which is venerable not by its duration, and which is not calculated by the number of years" (Minois, 1989, p.118). This interplay of the child within and the elder within is evident and felt by others when an older person exhibits elder expression.

Elders and Children are Look-alikes

In my work with older people who are admired and with children whom I adore, I have found that elderhood and childhood have these qualities in common. Both;

- Are impetuous
- Have a feel for dirt, clouds, birds and the sounds of nature
- Are egocentric (revived in the elder, natural to the child)
- Have a lack of concern with social convention
- Wear purple clothes, Santa Claus and/or ballerina outfits

- Have an awareness of the games people play to avoid intimacy
- Remember they are naturally creative and imaginative
- Are a problem for others
- Are contemplative of the unknown with little fear
- Have comfort with the mystery

There are life experiences that draw us out of our head and into our bodies and thence, into wonder. It is these kinds of experiences that connect us to our childhood, to the child within. If we watch we will find elders and children both involved in many of these experiences. In the Creation Spirituality tradition there is a meditation that both causes us to "let go of art as production...and return to art as process, which is the spiritual experience that creativity is about" (Fox, 1983a, p.192). It is called, art-as-meditation. Half of the time that I was in class at the University of Creation Spirituality in Oakland, California, I was immersed in activity that helped me "leave my head", enter my body and find a more direct route to my spirit. Art-as-meditation activities include many of the same experiences that elders and children use to connect to the child within:

- singing
- acting
- painting
- gardening
- walking in the woods
- playing in the sand
- making people laugh
- dancing
- drumming
- walking by the sea
- touching and talking with animals
- being sensual

These experiences don't only take us into our bodies. They can be the route to enlightenment. When we transcend ourselves and become simple, we become, or become again, children of God. The final place we reach in life may not be a pinnacle but rather a simplification that is childlike. I found this to some degree in a famous children's book.

Heidi and the Alm-Uncle

In the interplay between five-year-old Heidi and her seventy-year-old grandfather we find the synergy that makes life better both for the young and for the old. The book, *Heidi*, written by Joanna Spyri in 19th Century Switzerland, is a children's book. Yet, I find that a review of the story is one kind of preparation for elderhood. As I review parts of the book, watch for the magic that comes out of the experience of the old man being in the life of the young child. Watch for the permission to come to life that the child receives in the presence of the elder. Watch for how each expresses a fullness of being because neither is isolated and both are appreciated and respected by the other. You might ask yourself, does this children's book speak to us even though we are citizens of the second half of life? Could it speak to us more if we were more childlike?

The grandfather, who is called "Alm-Uncle" by the people in his family and in the small Swiss village of Dorfli, is compelled to bring Heidi into his home because she has been orphaned. He has been cut off from his extended family for years and, therefore, did not volunteer to care for his only granddaughter. He has lived far up Alm Mountain alone, bitter and angry about losses in his life he has not yet chosen to grieve. Heidi has been "dumped" by her aunt who has taken care of her since she was orphaned at age one. The aunt has fostered the child out of a sense of obligation but lacks passion for the duty. She persuades Alm-Uncle to take over by projecting on him guilt. He grumbles his way into the duty much like elderly people the world wide have done. His motivation at the beginning is not generativity as it could have been if he had responded to his granddaughter in the manner of an elder. He grudgingly moves Heidi into his small cabin, he tells her to sleep in the loft on a mound of hay.

"Bring your bundle of clothes," he said as he entered.

"I shan't want them anymore," replied Heidi.

"Why won't you need them anymore?" he asked aloud.

"I'd rather go like the goats, with their swift little legs."

The child presents almost immediately her joy with and connection to Earth and the two goats the grandfather owns. He knows deep inside why she suggests running about with no clothes on, but his initial response to her is practical and rigid. Then, he considers her more closely and says,

Elders As Revived Child

"So you shall, but bring the things along," commanded the grandfather (Spyri, 1984, p.17). Heidi has already found common ground with the old man: a lack of concern with social convention.

Heidi established a friendship with the goat herder, Peter, and his blind grandmother. They live on the same mountain within walking distance from the Alm-Uncles cabin. Heidi is concerned immediately with the rundown condition of this poor family's home.

"Grandfather, tomorrow we must take the hammer and the big nails and fasten the shutter at the grandmother's house and drive a good many nails; for everything creaks and rattles there".

"We must? We must do so? Who told you that?" asked the grandfather.

"Nobody told me so; I know it without" relied Heidi, "for everything is loose and it makes the grandmother anxious and afraid when the wind blows and she can't sleep. She thinks: "Now everything will fall down on our heads. And nobody can make it light anymore for the [blind] grandmother! She doesn't know how anyone can. But you can surely, grandfather" (Spyri, p.47). To the child the opportunity to improve the life of another is a natural response. The grandfather had to be reminded that this was a way of sharing his gifts and being of service.

Scarcely had Heidi opened the door to Peter's hut and run into the room when the grandmother called out from her corner:

"Here comes the child! It is the child!" (Spyri, p.49)

The old woman spoke aloud the joy people feel when a loving child comes within their space. In time the frustrated grandfather will also not be able to resist celebrating the child.

After about a year together, the grandfather is challenged by extended family and by the village pastor concerning schooling for Heidi. He is not inclined to be a part of the community and has confidence that Heidi is doing well learning from the land and learning from him. The little girl is taken from him by her aunt and placed with a well-to-do family in the city where she is to be a companion to a chronically sick girl Heidi's age. Heidi does not want to leave the Alm. The grandfather's child has left him and his child within now has no one to play with.

"From that day on, the Alm-Uncle looked more ill-natured than ever when he came down and passed through Dorfli. He spoke to no one; and with his cheese basket on his back, his enormous staff in his hand...he looked threatening". Mistakenly, the townspeople "were agreed that it was fortunate that the child was able to escape; for they had seen how she hurried away as if she were afraid the old man was coming after her to bring her back (Spyri, p.61).

"With Heidi gone, grandfather turned angry and forlorn" (Spyri, p.148).

He had a choice. He could express his gentle child within or depend on his granddaughter to be his route to be childlike. He had not yet remembered that he had within him the capacity for being childlike. Heidi returned a few weeks later. The people with whom she had lived recognized how unhappy she was without her grandfather. Upon returning she said,

"But you see, grandfather, I could hardly bear to wait any longer to come home again to you, and I often thought I should smother, it choked me so..." Heidi reported (Spyri, p.148). So, just as grandfather needed Heidi as an advocate for his child within, Heidi needed her adoring adult grandfather in her life to allow her to face the world with confidence.

"During the night her grandfather left his couch at least ten times, climbed the ladder and listened carefully to see if Heidi was still asleep and was not restless, and looked at the window where the moon used to shine in on Heidi's bed, to see if the hay he had stuffed into it was still there, for the moon should be kept out henceforth" (Spyri, p.151). Grandfather was able to watch over his own child within because the girl was in his life. Each time he attended to her, he was really tending to the child that was within him as well.

"Surely, grandfather, even if the grandmother is not willing, you will give me all my money, so that I can give Peter a piece for a roll everyday and two on Sunday."

"But the bed, Heidi?" said the grandfather (Spyri, p.158)

Heidi had been given some money by the family with whom she had stayed. She, immediately, saw it as an opportunity to bring pleasure to someone else. Grandfather wanted her to have a real bed. However, he found his way to the elder within and said to her,

"The money is yours, do whatever pleases you; you can get bread for the grandmother with it for a long year" (Spyri, p.158).

The elder knew things of the heart surpassed the practical.

"It may be that the Alm-Uncle is not so bad as they say; you can see how carefully he held the little one by the hand" (Spyri, p.163). The elder within is a source of compassion and gentleness.

"Grandfather, you never looked so handsome before as you have today," said Heidi.

"Do you think so?" said her grandfather, smiling. "Well, you see Heidi, I feel happy because I am on good terms with people and at peace with God and man...The dear Lord was good to me when He sent you up the Alm" (Spyri, p.165). The child has become a route to the old man's spirit. The child within is a source of spirit.

Heidi can become, like the elder, a source of blessing. She has befriended another older man, a doctor who is to become another elder in her life. He lost a son and has had difficulty in his grief. Heidi, because of her childlike access to joy says to him, speaking for herself and not consciously as his mentor,

"Surely now the dear Lord knows some joy which is to come out of this by and by, so I must be still for a little and not run away from Him. Then all at once it will happen so that you will see quite clearly that the dear Lord had nothing but good in His mind all the time; but because you could not see it at first, and only had the terrible sorrow all the time before you, you thought it would always remain so" (Spyri, p.190).

The gems that come from the mouths of babes can sound like it came from the mouths of wise elders.

The blind and dependent grandmother who lives down the mountain is also elder like some days. Despite her frail and blinded condition she celebrates life. This is one reason why she and Heidi connect so well. Speaking to the grandfather, the grandmother says,

"My dear uncle, what a splendid situation you have! Many a king might envy you! How well my Heidi looks! Like a little June rose!" she continued, drawing the child to her... "How glorious it is everywhere about!..." The grandmother is aware, despite her blindness of the way both the grandfather and Heidi have flourished being in the world for one another.

Later in this book I will demonstrate that elders have a better balance of masculine and feminine energy. Heidi provides grandfather with an opportunity to grow, to grieve and to let go of his frustrations. This brings him more into his feminine side. Next, we see an example of how that can look in an elder man. The sick friend of Heidi's, Klara, has come, wheelchair and all, to visit on the mountain. Grandfather and Klara's "grandmamma" are discussing Klara's care. Grandfather says,

"'If we should put the little daughter in her accustomed chair now, it would be better for her; the traveling chair is a little hard,' he said; and, without waiting for anyone to assist him, at once lifted the little girl invalid gently in his strong arms out of the straw chair and placed her with the greatest of care in the soft seat. Then he laid the shawls over her knees and wrapped her feet as comfortably on the cushion as if he had done nothing else all his life but care for invalids who could not use their limbs. The grandmamma looked at him in the greatest astonishment" (Spyri, p.229).

Recall how elders, as they enter the Newest Age, once again become connected to Earth. Here, Heidi demonstrates the connection that is possible for children:

"Sitting under the fir trees, Heidi had just been telling again about the flowers up there [in the pasture] and the sunset and the fiery rocks, and then such longing seized her to go up there again that she suddenly jumped up and ran to her grandfather, who was sitting in his shop carving.

'O, grandfather,' she called out before she was at all near him, "Will you come with us up to the pasture tomorrow? It is so lovely up there now!'"(Spyri, p.247) Heidi consistently gave her grandfather permission to celebrate the beauty of the place where he lived.

"For awhile, the old man stood earnestly watching how, after the high mountaintops, the green hills began to shine golden, and then the dark shadows gently faded away from the valley and a rosy light flowed in, and both heights and depths gleamed in the morning gold. The sun was up" (Spyri, p.249).

Could it be that the elder cannot feel the sun, hear the birds and experience the awe of creation without a link to the child inside that he was when he began life and never really lost? "One could say that God is biased in favor of the young. When we experience God, we experience a return to our beginnings, a newness, a rebirth" (Fox,1983b,p.180). To connect to creation we might have to become a child. Jesus said something like that. In the Hindu tradition there is a word, *lila*, which means divine play, the play of creation, destruction and re-creation. "*Lila* may be the simplest thing there is—spontaneous, childish, disarming. But as we grow and experience the complexities of life, it may also be the most difficult...achievement imaginable" (Nachmanovitch, 1990, p.1).Recalling the feel of childhood and acting out of its energy is a return to our authentic selves.The elder has recovered the authentic self, reconnected with wholeness and, once again, is balanced.

Play and Creativity

To play is to bring into motion, to bring into action. Creativity is an ability to see and respond and make out of this insight something new. Both play and creativity can be instinctual. Play and creativity are very much alike:

- Play is our natural state
- Play is our need to turn off judgment
- Play is process, not product
- Play is the Divine spark
- Play comes from the unconscious where God plays
- Play transforms us
- Play is the rich inner life overflowing into our outer being

When the Divine spark of play is expressed in tangible form, such as a sand castle, a collage or a painting, the expression of the image affects not only the creator but also the viewer. A painting can move us to tears and laughter. An emotional response like this alters an individual's body chemistry, which in turn affects metabolic functioning. When the emotional response is positive and uplifting it releases healing endorphins into the bloodstream that boost the immune system, reduce or eliminate the stress response, and enhance metabolic functioning. All of this results in healing.

When an older person lets loose the inner child and plays, they can be healed. They can be understood by children. They can find themselves once again. The evolutionary value of play is that it makes us flexible. There is a deep voice inside us latent from earliest childhood. The challenges, compromises, intellectual growth and adventures of growing up can dampen the sound of that voice. "The child is the voice of our own inner knowing. The first language of this knowing is play...By reinterpreting reality and begetting novelty, we keep from becoming rigid" (Nachmanovitch, p.50). We older people need to find our first language again, loosen our grip and get back to our awe of creation. We are the celebrants!

One example of this is the behavior of the Red Hat Society. While visiting a friend in Tucson several years ago, the founder of the society, Sue Ellen, impulsively bought a bright red fedora at a thrift shop, for no other reason than that it was cheap and, she thought, quite dashing. A year or two later she read the poem "Warning" by Jenny Joseph, which depicts an older woman in purple clothing with a red hat. Sue Ellen felt an immediate kinship with Ms. Joseph. She decided that her birthday gift to a friend would be a vintage red hat and a copy of the poem. She had always enjoyed whimsical decorating ideas, so she thought the hat would look nice hanging on a hook next to the framed poem. The friend got so much enjoyment out of the hat and the poem that Sue Ellen gave the same gift to another friend, then another, then another.

One day it occurred to these friends that they were becoming a sort of "Red Hat Society" and that perhaps they should go out to tea... in full regalia. They decided they would find purple dresses which didn't go with their red hats to complete the poem's image. The tea was a success. Soon, each of them thought of another woman or two she wanted to include, and they bought more red hats. Their group swelled to 18, and they began to encourage other interested people to start their own chapters. One of their members passed along the idea to a friend of hers in Florida, and their first "sibling" group was born. There about 150 chapters in Oregon alone.

The Red Hat Society has no official rules, although they have some rather strong suggestions, the first of which is regarding red hat attire. Of course, to be a Red Hatter, one should wear a red hat and a clashing purple ensemble at all meetings to keep up the spirit and purpose of the organization. They also suggest rather strongly that women under 50 stick to the pink hat and lavender attire until their fiftieth birthday which is a focus of special celebration. They believe this adds an element of celebration to aging. The members think celebration of aging is invaluable to women in our society who have learned to dread aging and avoid it at all costs. They believe that aging should be something anticipated with excitement, not something to dread (Red Hat Society, 2005).

Through the creative process, elders can become both healthier and more responsive to those who need our wisdom and nurturing. Creativity makes us more resilient and more capable of dealing with the adversity of loss that inevitably becomes a greater challenge as we age. To be creative in later life models what is possible. We can help the young confront their fear of aging by showing them our creativity.

CHAPTER FIVE

Eldering As Maturity

I have come to know my spirituality in terms of connection to all, to the One and to the Universe. When I began my study of the archetype of elder I was beginning to clarify, at the same time, the nature of my spiritual path. This was not my intention but neither was it coincidental. Going within to tap the energy of the elder within our soul and psyche is one way to find our path to maturity. Going within to find our center and then trying, as often as possible, to express ourselves from this place is another path to maturity. I have embraced aspects of a spirituality that helps express my belief in the source of life, the force that mediates between the body and the soul and paradoxically between God and me.

Much of what I call my spirituality comes from the writings of Matthew Fox. What Fox teaches is a challenge to the Christian model of spirituality that began with the fall of the human race from God's grace in the Garden of Eden and the subsequent redemption made available through the work of Jesus Christ. "It is a dualistic model and a patriarchal one; it begins its theology with sin and original sin, and it generally ends with redemption...[it] does not teach...about the New Creation or creativity, about justice-making and social transformation, or about...the God of delight. It fails to teach love of the earth or care for the cosmos" (Fox, 1983b, p.11). At the core of Fox's Creation Spirituality are the four paths to spiritual growth discussed in Chapter I. They overlap considerably with the processes and philosophy of growth into elderhood and, therefore, can help explain why the spiritual aspect of fourfold balance (i.e. spiritual, intellectual, physical and psychological) is for me the major one.

To utilize wisdom on behalf of others, to understand our oneness with Earth, to be a source of blessing and to reach out as a mentor, we have to have attained some personal balance. The call to elder is heard best by those who have discovered some sense of why they exist, who have a functional level of spiritual, intellectual, psychological and physical health and who have matured. Eldering is, paradoxically, an expression of kinship that comes from both a mature hunger to give back and comes from a childlike need to be in the world with glee. William Yeats wrote,

> Through all the lying day of youth
> I waved my leaves and flowers in the sun.
> Perhaps now I may wither—
> Into the truth.

When I was at mid-life I was convinced that the most mature role we play is that of parent. Now, from the viewpoint of a man who has become a resource to my children as they parent, maturity takes on a new meaning. I am a man,

> ...who, through years of experience and accumulated wisdom, having seen the beauty of human existence and its degradations, having experienced the love of other human beings and known, as well, hatred and vengeance, now serenely and peacefully views human existence and strives for meaning and intelligibility. Now, less dependent than ever on the vicissitudes of time and space, and purified in the struggles of human existence, the aging person comes to grips with him/herself in an ever-deepening encounter of acceptance of who he/she is and how life should be lived (Curran, 1985, p.74).

The elder years are a time "to make a special offering to fellow humans through a deeper involvement in the worldly sphere" (Bianchi, 1982, p.220). To be elder like is to accept that grown-ups don't just spend their retirement income, play but avoid responsibility.

Maturity is full personal development. The mature older person who has elder qualities has ripeness and a fully aged quality like that of good wine that can be nourishing to others. The maturation process includes a social, biological, spiritual, psychological and chronological evolution. Each of us matures differently but we can be said to all have clocks within that call us to be "on time" for our age in our development. Our biological clock chimes three adult phases beginning with adolescence. Women have hormonal changes that bring about a biological mid-life. A deterioration of our physical bodies gives men and women information about the last phase, what we have always called, old age. We have come to learn that we can do something to change the impact of these biological challenges. Physical deterioration in old age, for instance, can be slowed by good diet and appropriate exercise.

Our "Social Clock shapes a person for society. It represents a culture's way of saying 'when'" (Kotre, 1990, p.39). In the USA and Canada, different social clocks exist side by side. Wide varieties of people in these countries have different time schedules on which they base their lives. These include when to have children (if any) and when to end your career (if ever).

Our "psychological clock" is immensely personal and unique to each person. It refers to our inner schedule for growth and development. For the older person development is less measurable. "Its especially difficult to create an overarching scheme of 'ages and stages' for the second half of life. Then, the Biological and Social Clocks are quieter, their programs less determinate" (Kotre, p.71). There are, however, aspects of elder expression that give us clues to what we could be like in the Newest Age if we want to embrace the archetype of elder. Maturity then, for those of us past mid-life, can be redefined utilizing the spiritual model of elder.

However, as I explored in Chapter Four, maturity for an elder includes a paradoxical revival of childlike ways. Maturity is reached when the child is revived within. Eldering's gentle and compassionate touch is made possible by the elder's ability to tap the energy of their child within. Elder like behavior includes a sense of awe with creation. It includes an abandon that rejects social convention. It is characterized in part by the special connection elders and children have. So, mature elder expression is facilitated both by childlike behavior that is recalled and by the wisdom that leads to the elder's respect for children around them. Anthropologist Margaret Mead witnessed that in most cultures, both primitive and modern, there were three stages of development for the mature elder. In her book *Culture and Commitment*, she wrote that in the first stage, as children, we listen to and learn from our elders. Then, in young adulthood, Mead found that people find stimulation and learning through observing their peers. And then, in later life, if we are balanced she reported, we listen to the young.

To express elder like behaviors, a person must access that part of them that is centered and calming. That place is near the heart. The more time a person spends there, the quicker they mature and grow. From this growth comes a passion for social justice, kinship with Earth and a general sense of generativity. The person who matures has qualities of stability and courage, which are qualities reflective of full personal development. Maturity includes having grown through most of life's stages, learning from each and becoming a model for the potential of full development spiritually, psychologically and intellectually. The maturation process can be gradual, peaceful and progressive and it never reaches an ending. "An elder is a person who is still growing, still a learner, still with potential and whose life continues to have within it promise for, and connection to the future" (Schachter-Shalomi, pp.14-15). The elder is an evolved person who increasingly learns as life gets longer that life has variations, that perspectives are numerous and that there is only one truth: all people are good. "Since 'blessing' is the theological word for 'goodness', original blessing is about original goodness" (Fox, 1983a, p.7) We were born into goodness.

Elders celebrate their family and enhance its functioning by being present and involved. This person then takes this blessing, which has opened their heart, and moves into the realm of parent where they teach the skills needed to move energetically into the world. Next, the maturing person formally separates from their parents, achieves mastery of what they have been taught and is now capable of mentoring others. They grow from adulthood into elderhood. If a mature person lives long enough, they revere life as a cherished gift. They develop a hunger to serve others while humbly understanding their limitations. This elder cultivates intimacy and has numerous friends.

The mature person is loyal to something greater than she is: a philosophy, country, leader, and family. She arouses excitement in others about her commitment to bettering her community, and poses a threat to the shadow forces that are devoted to the destruction of people and the environment. The mature person believes in their intuition. Children enjoy mature people because they are playful, compassionate, spiritual and gentle. Women enjoy the mature male because he is confident, nurturing, ordered and empathetic. Men enjoy mature women because they don't whine, have chosen the path of heart and "are fierce about what matters to them" (Bolen, 2003, p.47). Mature people see inner beauty. "This beauty lies deep within the self: no longer external, it cannot be taken away" (Fischer, 1995, p.10). Where the young man may first be taken by the youthful beauty of a woman, the man who is mature experiences an older woman as beautiful because he senses her spirit, her ability to connect at the heart and her depth. Be careful not to mix up the mature man with the typical older man. They are very different.

The Three Challenges

There are at least three life challenges that are only faced after we enter the time of our life when elderhood is possible. This usually occurs when we are in or near our sixties and in good health. The first challenge is to make the transition from your career to what follows. This challenge requires grieving, a letting go and the discovery of a new way of utilizing our creativity. In the second challenge, we must ask the question, "Do I wish to take my long life experience and utilize it on behalf of others?" We don't need to decide to be in service but we do need to ask the question. The third challenge is to face the challenge of life completion. In life completion we address end of life planning, explore what our legacy will be, confront the reality of our mortality and celebrate the source of life itself. The poet Rumi asked,

> Why does a date-palm lose its leaves in autumn?
> Why does every beautiful face grow in old age
> Wrinkled like the back of a Libyan lizard?
> Why does a full head of hair get bald?
> Why is the tall, straight figure
> That divided the ranks like a spear
> Now bent almost double?
> Why is it that the

Lion strength weakens to nothing?
The wrestler who could hold anyone down
Is led out with two people supporting him,
Their shoulders under his arms?
God answers,
"They put on borrowed robes
And pretend they were theirs.
I take the beautiful clothes back,
So that you will learn the robe
Of appearance is only a loan."
Your lamp was lit from another lamp.
All God wants is your gratitude for that.

The mantle of elderhood in the mature person replaces the mantle of youth. God takes back "the beautiful clothes" when we become young-old (i.e., over sixty-five and healthy) as a reminder that our beauty has always come from a deep place within, "another lamp". It is only after the clothes are taken back that we can, once again, see this clearly. For me, the life challenges of transition into elderhood, of service and of life completion are gifts of the spirit. Developing maturity is a spiritual process.

The Industrial Era and Immaturity

Those who have been victims of the unloving and dangerous acts of men have experienced the impact of immature men. They are men who live in men's bodies but experience life like a boy. This incongruence is confusing at best, spiritually destructive at worst. As people age, they will ideally mature, but absent that growth, their soul begins to disintegrate and they live in fear. "The individual unit of evolution is the soul" (Zukav, 1989, p.186). As a person comes to experience creativity, healing and love, he lives off the energy of the soul. "When the energy of the soul is recognized, acknowledged and valued, it begins to infuse the life of the personality" (Zukav, p.31). Soul is the experience of God and it is the place in a person that connects us to all people.

The Great Depression created a loss of soul as well as property and income. Our hunger for wages and profit left us vulnerable to a great emotional depression as our grandparents lost their jobs in the 1930's. The

Great Crash of the stock market was devastating because the successful business people were "machine men" finding personal meaning in producing wealth. European farmers just prior to the Industrial Revolution of the 18th century worked about 1,600 hours annually, less than half the 3,650 hours worked each year by the average American worker in 1850 and less than the 2,050 hours worked annually by American workers today (Schor, 1992, p.45). Women and children worked as well. In fact, as late as 1820, children comprised more than two-thirds of the workers in numbers of textile mills in the New England states of the USA. The majority of workers in the USA textile industry of the 19th Century were young women (Dublin, 1979, p.16). However, by 1900 most women worked in the home and most men worked in agriculture. By 1860 the proportion of the work force employed outside of agriculture, however, decreased from 40 percent to less than 30 percent in 1820.

The elder who finds their pathway usually has teachers, mentors or models to admire. Prior to the advent of machinery, older crafts people provided mentorship to their apprentices. Many young men and women learned a trade from their parents because the family worked together on the farm or within the village commons. 18th Century people were not very mobile. Life usually began and ended in the same community. On the village common a child could find mentors of many kinds: aunts; neighbors; village merchants; grandparents; and parents. Men and women expected to teach the young. Their close proximity and lack of mobility enhanced their accessibility. Children assumed that older people would be mentors.

Since the 19th Century restructuring of society, we have redefined the roles of men and women. In industrializing the culture, we not only enclosed workers in the factories but left most women overwhelmed with homebound duty. In pre-industrial times and for centuries prior, the village commons were the primary social units of England. All but the royalty, landed gentry, military and church hierarchy lived on the land and tilled it for subsistence. Those who farmed held land as shareholders, making community decisions democratically.

Pre-industrial era nuclear families worked side by side. Much of the work was assigned by sex. The assumed work roles of men and women varied from country to country, but it was common, for example, that men often planted while women harvested. Children could copy their fathers and mothers because they were both present. Then came the Enclosure Acts in Great Britain that literally separated people from their land. The government supported the goals of the large landowners who were the taxpayers: to fence off land worked by the people and create more space to raise sheep. The economic activities that justified the Enclosure Acts dislodged those who worked the land from the land. The Industrial Revolution completed the process of enclosing the worker out of the home and into the workplace. "The immediate effect of the Industrial Revolution upon the countries to which it came, was to cause a vast, distressful shifting and stirring of the mute, uneducated, leaderless, and now more and more property less common population" (Wells, 1920, p.656). This "shifting and stirring" began a process that left men's souls undernourished. This social and economic movement of people destroyed communities, created uncounted numbers of economic refugees and disrupted the norms for living of all those it affected.

The shattering of souls began with the forced movement of people from the land and was compounded by the Industrial Revolution two centuries later. When the larger landowners began to build fences to enclose their land and their stock, they also cut off people from their natural interplay with Earth. Being in the land stirs a sense of kinship, an honoring of the source of life and an understanding of fertility that is understood by the elder earthkeeper. Earthkeepers celebrate fertility both on the land and in the people. What began in the 19th Century was an impoverishment—the opposite of fertility and generativity. To be impoverished is to have exhausted fertility and the inclination to kinship with Earth. The impoverished approach life with fear and desperation. People were forced to act from a place in their psyche that is survival focused, logical and causes little emotional expression. Since the source of elder energy is at our center limited access to soul and psyche limits our ability to express ourselves in an elder way. People moved away from their heart center when they left the land and the family. Their sense of mental, physical, psychological and spiritual balance was diminished in this move.

A Revolution of the Spirit

In the 1960's, women challenged the then "feminine mystique" that had been reinforced by the business world's preference for male leadership. There had been female voices advocating for women even during the Industrial Era. Most notably, Mary Wollstonecraft wrote *Vindication of the Rights of Women* crying out about the unfair influence of men (Encyclopedia Britannica, 2004). The Industrial Revolution was also the beginning of a feminist consciousness. Women were not as willing to submit to the domestic plan that had evolved and was so dramatically demonstrated in the patriarchal Industrial Era. They resented patriarchy: a social and political system where the eldest males believed they were superior to women. Socially aware women wanted men to understand that women were their equal. At issue was in part men's sense of personal power. Men had lost touch with how a person plays an effective part in the community and in the family. They had isolated themselves in the new work place. By 1976 feminists such as Adrienne Rich wrote that, "...a pervasive recognition is developing that the patriarchal system cannot answer for itself; that it is not inevitable; that it is transitory; and that the cross-cultural, global domination of women by men can no longer be either denied or defended" (Rich, 1976, p.32). This had become public rhetoric for the first time since the establishment of patriarchy nearly 5000 years earlier.

The experience of power over has led into inaccurate assumptions about men's power, however. For instance, as a small group of men perpetuate domestic violence, the overall impact of violent crime is on men, not only by men. Men are three times more likely than women to be victims of murder and twice as likely to be victims of other violent crimes. Over the past 40 years the cancer death rate for men has increased 21 percent while the rate for women has remained the same. Men represented 55% of the work force in 1990 but 93% of all job-related deaths (Kimbrell, 1995, p.5). Increasingly powerless men have become very vulnerable.

Power is also defined in terms of money and property. A masculine mystique surrounding our fear of men has developed that includes the belief that men have more of both money and property. The U.S. Dept. of Commerce, Bureau of the Census tells us that women's financial worth is considerably higher than men's. With men living shorter lives, women are left with the wealth. Women also have greater spending power and lower spending obligations (Farrell, 1993, p.33). This is not to say women are the problem. Women are filling gaps left by men who leave the home, rush head-long after power for power's sake and die too young. The men end up with enough stress to detach emotionally and not enough health to avoid deadly illness.

The U.S. Department of Labor reported in 1995 that about one million men in their prime working years had stopped looking for jobs. Not only are many just sitting home, but also in 1995 dollars, the weekly wage of those males working has dropped from $611 in 1979 to $538 in 1995. Women, meanwhile, have been increasing their activity in the workforce and their average wage has been increasing. Women have been less impacted by the loss of manufacturing jobs to low-wage countries and white-collar jobs being replaced by computers. Women are even less affected by affirmative action policy.

I suppose you could say that being male can be discouraging. Boys are twice as likely as girls to suffer from autism and eight times more likely to be treated for hyperactivity. Two-thirds of special education is devoted to boys and over 60 percent of high school dropouts are male. More women graduate from college than do men. It is estimated that 270,000 of our veterans are homeless and that 70% of the homeless are single men. Men's economic and political power is at risk in light of these facts (Kimbrell, 1995, pp.3-13).

Men are torn between their commitment to provide and their desire to be emotionally attached to those they love. Nearly 80 percent of married men with preschool children are employed full-time. Half of all marriages disintegrate with men receiving custody of the children in less than 20 percent of contested divorce actions. One out of five divorced fathers sees his children as little as once a year. One out of every two sees his children only several times a year (Popenoe, 1996, p.31). Men have lost hope about their role in parenting. Finding time in their work-a-day lives to be with their families is difficult.

The impoverished male of today demonstrates how it looks to be fragmented with "various parts of his personality...split off from each other and leading...independent and often chaotic lives... He remains a boy, not because he wants to, but because no one has shown him the way to transform his boy energy into man energies" (Moore, 1990, p.90). The person who abuses their children, the politician who takes advantage of their constituency, the minister who hates homosexuals, the gang-banger who inflicts pain, the absent parent and the tyrant boss all have one thing in common. They are all spiritually impoverished which results in a non-nurturing, unemotional and selfish sense of being.

Control and balance come with maturity. Immature, spiritually impoverished people often operate out of the "shadow side" of their psyche. The shadow usually contains inferior qualities that are balanced only by a good self-esteem. If we don't remain conscious of the power of our shadow, our dark side, it can lead us in an unhappy if not destructive direction. The immature are out of balance and they respond too willingly to shadow energy. The insensitive, fearful energy in the psyche of a person who is acting immaturely is running their life. "The Shadow Warrior carries into adulthood that adolescent insecurity, violent emotionalism and desperation of the [archetypal] Hero" (Moore, 1990, p.90). The archetypal energy of the underdeveloped Warrior interferes with intimacy. Immature men have let loose the Shadow Warrior.

I was raised in the 40s and 50s by parents who grew into adulthood in the Depression. My grandparents, who also lived in the time of transition from rural to industrial America, raised our parents. My grandparents and parents were focused on earning a living and obtaining wealth. Their ancestors had been in the land and were driven by a desire to survive. My father was a victim of the separation of people from the land and the subsequent change into the lifestyle of a wage earner. Over the last couple of centuries, wage earners have been preoccupied with earning an income. Before the enclosure of men into the workplace, men worked to survive and to express creativity. In striving for the fruits of their labor, Industrial Era workers lost touch with the harvest of self and the spirit. Because our fathers had lost touch with their center, their soul, they failed to model maturity. Modern men's access to mature energy in the psyche has been reduced by this tragic reality.

I was among many children who lacked the mentoring needed to show us how to access mature energy within ourselves. My mother's influence was greater than my father's because, like most the men, he was emotionally detached from the family because of his work. Following our mothers, the only available parent, has led, paradoxically, too many young men to "put down their swords". We forgot at that point that although it can be dangerous, the use of the sword by a mature man is motivating, invigorating and positive. The revolution led by women in the 1960's began not only a movement toward an egalitarian spirit; it reintroduced the mature concept of masculine-feminine balance. What has come from this time is a greater confidence in a partnership model of society and a gradual movement away from a *dominator* model such as the models based on immature expression called *patriarchy and matriarchy* (Eisler, 1995, p.xvii).

Immaturity at Work

As an employee assistance professional, I witnessed immaturity in the workplace from a unique perspective. An employee assistance counselor assists people at work to prevent and treat mental health and other personal problems. In this work, I saw how immaturity led to an imbalance of a person's mental condition. People at work in business and industry, especially those aspiring to management, have less time with their families. They also have increased pressure to compete, which can lead to a hunger for status and power, a guarded interpersonal style, a fear of termination and a belief that wealth and status is the measure of their worth. I am as good an example as any.

I was the chief executive officer and founder of my consulting firm. Carrying this title satisfied my need for control over my life. I was not just the elder of our company, or the owner, but also the CEO! The challenge for me was to separate the power I had from the power-over I had. On the occasions that I was aware of my personal power, I experienced it as influence, but it was often generative. I felt like an elder at these times. If I wielded my status, my power as power over, I lost a connection to the people who worked for me. I lost their cooperation. The more cooperation I facilitated, the more we all accomplished.

Spiritless bullies want power-over others. When I operate from fear, from my "inner coward", I want power-over others because I want to control the situation. Adults who are immature are often in charge at work, but they are paradoxically powerless. Their influence ends when the employee goes home. While employees are at work, they are putting up with the immature boss, not supporting her or working toward consensus. Men like me are products of an industrial world. Those inclined to be involved in activity that nourishes the soul are constantly dancing with maintaining the balance between personal power and power-over, competition and cooperation, and fear and love. There are too many incidents of immaturity in the workplace. The workplace expression of immaturity has led, for example, to the need for nondiscrimination policies in most companies. In the modern workplace we need rules to discourage sexual harassment. Policies are written on how to cope with violence at work as well as drug abuse at work.

Pre-modern people worked so that they could have food and shelter. Their work was a natural response to basic needs such as survival and hunger. Then, later on in history, it was discovered that "things", once created by work, could be traded. Trading allowed for needs to be met without working. So the drive to satisfy basic needs led to work which, in turn, led to the creation of goods that could be either used or traded. Artists showed us that some things could be created for their own sake. We also created things for their own sake that could be counted and accumulated. We discovered that we could accumulate more than other people could and that the other people envied us. The accumulation of lots of envied things led to the admiration of wealth. Somewhere between creating things for their own sake and creating wealth, some of us lost touch with our soul. Accumulating is fine until it becomes more important than the reason a person exists on Earth.

The Machines

In the Industrial Era, people figured out how to create things faster by using machines. Once we created machines, we recreated our image of ourselves. "As we cast, soldered, burned and molded the ore and fossil fuels of the Earth to fashion the great engines of the industrial age, these machines just as surely recast and remolded modern consciousness" (Moore, 1990, p.90). Modern people's work and play are concerned with integrating machines into our life. Machines like televisions, computers and telephones are required for all who can afford them. We learn with machines. We communicate with machines. We travel with machines. We process our thoughts with machines. However, the image of personhood we developed is like the image we have of machines.

Depending on machines can turn people into machines. To the machine man even sexuality becomes a technical skill. The male lover becomes a "love machine". The machine man "becomes part of the total machinery that he controls and is simultaneously controlled by. He has no plan or goal in life, except doing what the logic of technique determines him to do...Robots are among the greatest achievement of his technical mind, and some specialists assure us that the robot will hardly be distinguished from living men" (Kimbrell, 1995, p.46). People who become machine-like are efficient problem solvers, who bring home the bacon, which is proof of our productive nature. We are in control and rational and, most of all, efficient. The most longed for trait of a good machine is efficiency. To compete successfully, we need to work long hours with little attention given to our health. The most profound impact the machine man model has on us is to starve the soul. Machine-like people are more like replaceable parts than passionate beings. They are expendable. It used to be that only the male machines were sent to war. Now females can be in the military and allowed to die on purpose.

Competition

Another commitment people made as they became producers in the industrialized and mechanized world of work was to compete — to compete for jobs, the best pay, the most success and the highest level of job assignment. Competition both binds and divides us. This nearly uncontrollable process goes on in corporate conference rooms as well as at "new age" gatherings. According to Goldberg, in the mind of the competitor, taking a sick day away from the "grind" means:

- His or her territory is threatened and someone might usurp his position
- Someone might discover they really aren't needed or might try to replace them
- Each day in bed is money lost
- She's not a capable warrior and doesn't hold up under pressure (Goldberg, 1976, p.105)

In competition, the questions are: Who's winning? How much was their bonus? Who wants to go first? Most competitors remember the humiliation they felt when they weren't successful on the playground or athletic field. We jokingly report, "Yeah, I never got picked." Only a small number of people win a lot of the time. Competition, of course, is not an experience in intimacy. "We are told that real men don't ask for help but only the 'opportunity' to compete...As competition becomes the male's main avenue of self-validation, fear of losing in competition remains the single greatest anxiety for many men" (Kimbrell, 1995, p.74) Even with similar abilities, people oriented toward mastery and hard work typically achieve more if they avoid competing. Competition in business and sports can lead to better services, new products and higher scores. There are, however, psychological hazards to competition. Competition is the opposite of cooperation. "Healthy competition" can be a contradiction. Competition often leads to insecurity, anxiety, jealousy and hostility.

Men Do, Women Be

Since the 1950's, many sociologists and psychologists have agreed with the instrumental/expressive divide between men and women. This is a product of the belief that men are primarily oriented toward activity, achievement and power. Women are believed to be oriented toward nurturance and relationship (Silverstein, 1994, p.30). The immature male, he who reinforces the masculine mystique, risks getting lost while seeking achievement and power. He gets lost in "doing"! Warren Farrell said, "women are human beings. Men are humans doing" (Farrell, 1993, p.33) In maturity, on the other hand, achievement and power are integrated with a hunger for cooperation, mastery and intimacy. It is a blessing that men are oriented differently than women, hence, the wonderful energy that is created when men and women interplay. Kimura says in her book, it is likely that men and women are literally hard-wired in different ways (Kimura, 1992, p.119).

Perhaps gender differences are also culturally influenced, however. One of the most infamous examples is the impact of replacing the farm with the factory. The workplace valued instrumental qualities that men have such as their better-developed spatial view. Home life requires expressive qualities such as those of the nurturing specialists—women.

The Industrial Revolution was so powerful culturally that it restyled the meaning of manhood and womanhood. This era enforced the position of women locked into the home. "Until the turn of the twentieth century, domestic service remained the largest occupation of female labor" (Dublin, 1979, p.13). This isn't the whole story. As early as 1835, for instance, women played an active role in the growth of the labor movement in the USA. Men and women were gradually drawn into the corporate world over two centuries. It gradually tore the fabric of accepted masculine and feminine expression. It left behind distortions in the masculine and feminine archetypes we are familiar with today.

Historically men have showed an inclination to at least three functions in most societies: protector, provider and teacher. Since industrialization women have been increasingly interested in playing these male roles. Men are less needed, therefore, in their historical roles and are being asked to participate more in childrearing and other domestic pursuits.

In much of the pre-industrial world a clearer standard of manhood prevailed. To be fulfilled as a man, an adult male, if firstborn, took ownership of the family land from his father, headed a household and carefully guided the destiny of his children (Rotundo, 1985, pp.7-25). However, the enclosure of men out of the home gradually placed women in a preeminent household role. The 20th Century rejection of the Calvinist notion of innate child depravity made reasonable the shifting of children's care to the maternal, less instrumental parent.

Despite its patriarchal qualities, what we now call the "nuclear family" represented for women a significant advance over their situation in the pre-industrial family. Throughout the 19th Century more women married, bore children who survived and had husbands who lived jointly with them. The 19th Century Victorian family became more of a partnership than a hierarchy. Male authority became symbolic as respect for women grew and mothers began to develop domestic influence (Popenoe, 1996, p.12). Around 1800 in England female political unions were formed and, in time, became religious and charitable institutions managed by women. However, a "nostalgia for lost status [came with] the assertion of newfound rights...the woman's status turned upon her success as a housewife in the family economy, in domestic management...baking and brewing, cleanliness and child-care." Women's new independence, in the mill was felt simultaneously as a loss in status and in personal independence. "...they looked back to a "golden" past in which home earnings from spinning...and the like, could be gained around their own door. In good times the domestic economy...supported a way of life centered upon the home" (Thompson, 1963, p.55). Each stage in industrial specialization struck at the family's function disturbing customary relations between husband and wife, parents and children, and differentiating more sharply between "work" and "life".

The shift in the definition of masculinity away from protector and provider toward self-aggrandizing individualist resulted in the diminished influence of fathers. Male interest in a new expression drew men together in groups. Fraternal orders began to grow in the late 19th Century. The humor of men in these clubs was disparaging of marriage, the dominance of women and family responsibilities. In reaction, women and children began to buy the masculine mystique. Males, including fathers, were viewed as inherently suspect and the work world was felt to pose the threat of tempting fathers away from the home. "From being considered a central, natural and unproblematic aspect of being a man, as it had been with the Puritans, fatherhood became something which needed to be promoted by the culture" (Demos, 1986, p.55). Today, numerous social scientists suggest that the father is no longer necessary to the economic survival of the family.

The early factories were disordered and unstable. Workers were destabilized and it made them vulnerable to vices and other less than civilized behaviors. Personal integrity was largely discounted in the work place of the 19th Century. "The men who lived and worked in this environment were necessarily imperiled and maleness itself seemed to carry a certain odor of contamination" (Demos, 1986, p.55). Today we have families that feel isolated from relatives and their surrounding community. The burden of parenting has increasingly fallen to the nuclear family. At the same time, the nuclear family is disintegrating. Up until the cultural changes of the 1960s and 1970s both fathers and mothers were considered by most social scientists as core to the healthy growth of children and said "no child should be brought into the world without a man assuming the role of father, the male link between the child and the rest of the community" (Malinowski, 1962, p.63). Today we debate whether children need a man's full time influence as they grow.

As a father of six, I applaud much of the vision of the New Father coming out of the prepared childbirth movement. Who doesn't admire hands-on, involved fatherhood? However, the most admirable theme of the New Father model: the celebration of men to act tenderly toward their children is not new at all. 18th Century philosopher Jean-Jacques Rousseau said, in speaking about the family, that "The habit of living together gave rise to the sweetest sentiments known to men: conjugal love and paternal love." The New Father reminds us that some men are following their intuition to be complete human beings. Men prompted by soul derive pleasure from their connection to men and women, and openly and spontaneously share their feelings and dreams. The New Father personalizes rather than objectifies relationships and parenting means responding to the cues of his children. Older men who, as young fathers, embraced the call to "new fathering" will have a special insight into the nurturing role of elder.

The elder is an advocate for the young and believes that advocacy for youth means being aware of a new psychology for men and women. This mind-set is another way of defining maturity. Maturity does not incorporate the juvenile or underdeveloped aspects of being that have led to destructive behavior such as the devaluation of women or a hunger for power for its own sake. These are examples of immaturity and they are the unfortunate but predictable result of the gender role socialization process unique to the beginning of the Industrial Revolution.

CHAPTER SIX

Becoming An Elder

*T**he process of becoming an elder requires that a person seek to express qualities of elderhood.* Elderhood is not a goal or state of being that, once reached, requires no further striving. Elder like people make errors, have embarrassing moments, experience grief and loss and yet can, on a good day, be an extraordinary natural resource. Best of all they know how to access their elder energy and embrace the stage of life called elderhood. There are three processes that encourage growth into elderhood, and we will review each in this chapter.

The first is to recognize and embrace the fact that elderhood is a stage of development. The second is initiation into elderhood. The third and most complex is to do the intellectual, psychological, physical and spiritual personal work necessary to grow into elderhood. The person who expresses elderhood is doing something needed for their community. They share their wisdom in an active way. And they continue to grow and learn in a way only possible through the give and take of generative relationships.

The man or woman who expresses elder like behaviors maintains a connection to those who would gain from their elderhood. They are interesting, energizing and passionate people. Their behavior inspires young people who become drawn to them. The aspiring elder must first find their elder energy and learn how to bring it forward and allow it to influence their behavior. Then, once being recognized by the young or any persons they serve, the elder can do the work necessary to grow up and act like an elder.

Elderhood As A Stage of Personal Growth

Some poets, psychologists and anthropologists have recognized that there are predictable stages of human development that include elder expression. They are a way of describing a developmental theory. The developmental theory we are reviewing here describes change over a lifetime in "areas of behavior or psychological activity, such as thought, language, social behavior, or perception" (Miller, 1989, p.6). Proponents call it different names, but in poetry, psychology and social anthropology, stages of personal growth can be found that are celebrated. They include a generative, spiritual maturity in the second half of life. I call this stage elderhood. Let's consider four models of personal growth that suggest strongly that elderhood happens naturally if we allow it to become a part of our growth into maturity.

Erikson

Erik Erikson MD asserted in 1950 that there are eight steps in adapting psychologically and socially to life. Erikson put forth his eight stages of human development in 1950 (Erikson, 1950, pp.247-275). There are other psychologists and educators who suggest that we can identify stages of cognitive and moral development as well, but no better description of the psychological developmental process has been offered since Erikson. Research done since Erikson popularized developmental theory has shown that adult life does not necessarily progress through fixed, predictable steps. Erikson's work provides, however, a perspective that has earned common acceptance. Each stage is characterized by a "crisis" that must be resolved for healthy development to occur. I believe that some of Erikson's crises stir a call to elderhood in a person. I have identified these crises below in **bold**.

Erikson's Stages
1. First year of life   Crisis: Trust versus Mistrust
2. Toddler   Crisis: Autonomy vs. Shame and Guilt
3. Preschooler   Crisis: Initiative vs. Guilt
4. School age   Crisis: Competence vs. Inferiority
5. Adolescence   Crisis: Identity vs. Role Confusion
6. Young adulthood   Crisis: Intimacy vs. Isolation

7. Adulthood   Crisis: **Generativity** vs. Stagnation
8. Maturity   Crisis: **Ego Integrity** vs. Despair

Stage theories suggest that there are passages people must traverse in life. As we review a few of the stage theories, keep in mind that development is neither finished nor easily put into a formula. The crisis of one stage may reawaken during another stage. Identity crises such as the struggle between autonomy and shame, for example, are not only present in adolescence. The development of competence is a dynamic process that occurs throughout life and not just in Erikson's fourth stage. Children develop because of biological changes dictated by genetics as well as psychosocial forces. However, environmental and social forces have more impact on adult development because older people are no longer growing physically.

More important than the specific stages within a theory are the social, spiritual, intellectual and psychological challenges we face as we mature. Erikson believed these challenges included in particular, generativity and ego integrity, for people living into the second half of life. "Ego integrity ...implies an emotional integration which permits participation by follower ship as well as acceptance of the responsibility of leadership" (Erikson, p.269). He took the word "generative", which means the power to generate, and popularized it as the noun "generativity". He said that his stages consisted mostly of youth passages, but had his theory been focused on adulthood, "generativity" would have been his central issue. Generativity is a quality that makes people into parents, teachers, mentors and creative and learning creatures. Anything, anyone who facilitates the growth of something living is generative.

Retirement

The American attitude about the second half of life leads us to a preoccupation with retirement which can be contradictory to a generative expression. The paradox here is that this worker's dream of the future focuses mostly on retreating, not generating! In our move to "retire", we can be seen to pull away from younger people and the community. If we are healthy and have the financial capability to do so, most of us want to simplify our lives after age 65 and enjoy the fruits of decades of work for wages. However, our work world structured our time, was a major source of social connection and provided for many of us our primary sense of purpose. Mature adults experiencing despair about physical depletion, a loss of purpose, a community bias toward aging and a reduction in personal potency face a paradox. The despair leads to the belief that life is too short to start another life consisting of mentoring, teaching and sharing the wisdom gained from long life experience. In premodern times retirement had no meaning. The concept grew out of the Industrial Era.

Maybe there is a way to enter life's later stages, celebrate our release from the demands of regular work hours and still find a way to grow into elderhood. Generativity is a concern for supporting and guiding the next generation. What life style nourishes the soul? Does it include travel, golf, fishing, a new business venture, or painting? For the upper middle class in Western societies, of course it does. However, we must accept responsibility for not having shared our wisdom if these activities cause us to loose contact with the younger generation who could flourish with an elder in their life. To become a resource to others, we must be accessible. If our second-half-of-life activities make us inaccessible either physically or emotionally, we have missed an opportunity for service. How do those who would receive our legacy see us? How confident are they that we have wisdom? Can we demonstrate our passion for eldering by being inaccessible either geographically or by an attitude of isolation?

In the final stage of life, older adult's can either consider life meaningful or despair about goals not reached. To accomplish ego integrity, older people must accomplish all of the following according to developmental theories:

- develop trust, autonomy and independence
- show initiative
- remain industrious
- have a definable identity
- seek affiliation
- accept their mortality
- seed the young with good ideas.

In previous chapters we considered the devastating impact of industrialization and a spiritual "impoverishment" of men and women. Impoverishment is the opposite of fertility and generativity. Industrialized people lost touch with the land, with the family and, therefore, lost touch with the catalysts to growth into maturity. Human beings need the ability to confront, struggle with and advance through stages of growth—the "passages". Retirement comes at the time of life when four major life challenges face us. First we must grieve the end of our work life. A two or three year process of transitioning into the time after we stop the way we working at mid-life is common to many. Second, I suggest we need to decide whether we want to move into the community as an elder resource after doing the necessary personal work to tap our elder energy. Third, we need a plan for utilizing the 15-30 year period of creative life ahead that was not available to our grandparents. Finally, but not until we are nearly into our 90s, we can engage the "golden years" that we were led to believe by retirement myths came shortly after we quit work. The task of this time is life completion.

Bly

In poet Robert Bly's controversial book, *Iron John*, the author addresses the effect of losing touch with our roots and the family traditions that facilitate growth. The book is a resurrection of a fairy tale in which a mentor guides a young man through eight stages of growth unique to men. Being off the land and in the city seeking wealth, men in the 19th Century began to lose touch with their mentors. These mentors were primarily the fathers and grandfathers the factory workers had left behind on family farms. Bly mourns the impoverishment that resulted from losing contact with our fathers, both geographically and emotionally. He hungers for male initiation rites that were more common in the pre-industrial world. The eight stages of life Bly offers can be found in various myths throughout history. It is interesting that all the stage theorists reviewed in this chapter count seven or eight stages of growth whether they have studied poetry, myth, psychology, anthropology or the customs of indigenous cultures. Once again, I have highlighted in bold below those stages that most apply in the second half of life.

Bly's Stages
1. Early childhood   Task: Bonding with Mother
2. Late childhood   Task: Leaving the Mother
3. Early adolescence   Task: Bonding with Father

4. Late adolescence	Task: Leaving the Father
5. Early adulthood	Task: The Quest
6. Young adulthood	Task: **Working with the Mentor**
7. Adulthood	Task: **Apprenticeship**
8. Maturity	Task: **Integration of the Masculine and the Feminine within**

Bly is concerned primarily with the development of gender identity and the expression of masculine and feminine energy found in our psyche. We are born of the mother and nourished by her feminine passion for nourishing, enfolding and shielding the child. The study of maternal-infant bonding has shown that when a child and his mother bond physically and psychologically, the child's future is more likely to include blessings such as good health, high IQ and good social skills (Klaus, 1976, p.10). The challenge in early childhood is to connect with the nurturing power of our feminine parent. Erikson would call this a major "trust" experience.

Next, a boy must leave the energy field of the mother and seek balance in the power of the masculine. In Bly's story, the mother keeps the key to the masculine. To access the power of the masculine, a child needs to come to his father through his mother, leaving her and taking the key to the cage that houses Iron John, the masculine aspect of a boy's soul. The challenge in the second stage of both Erikson's and Bly's models is to risk autonomy and bond with the father who models initiative and aggression.

The increasing problems of fatherlessness and out-of-wedlock births in North America deprive young boys and girls of the opportunity to experience a male model. If our fathers cannot give us what we need to access the masculine in ourselves, we can get stuck in immaturity. An answer to this dilemma is male elderhood. In ancient times the older men would teach the younger men how to become healthy men. In today's world, mature older men could fill this role if they were accessible and willing to serve as a mentor.

In Bly's model, the developing male must eventually leave the sphere of the father as well as the mother. If an older mature man did not play the role of father in a child's life, he can at least assist a boy's development by playing a role in life's apprenticeship. Mentors are essential to the developing person's growth into self-identity and competence as "his own person". An apprentice is a learner. The ideal advocate or model for the apprentice is not usually a parent but rather a more objective older person. This is an excellent opportunity for the person wanting to express elder energy. In Pat Conroy's novel, *Beach Music*, we find this description of one boy's mentor:

> Jordan turned his blue eyes at the drawling, overweight coach who ran a gas station for a living and brought an irrepressible love of sport and young boys to the task of coaching...Jordan saw the goodness of the man below the primitive, fascist exterior that is the general rule among the southern fraternity of coaches. It was the man's basic and abiding sweetness that Jordan felt as coach Langford put the ball back into Jordan's glove and said, "Son, now I'd like to see you strike him out" (Conroy, 1995, p.123).

In Erikson's model, completing the development of a mature self requires an experience of intimacy, generativity, and finally, balance (what he calls "ego integrity"). Bly would have us reach these goals through a complete enfolding of both the masculine and feminine energy in our psyche. Men and women often express intimacy and generativity differently. Many men are energized when expressing these qualities. They are a source of peace and serenity when expressed by men or women.

The man in *Iron John* was about 50 years old when he reached the last developmental stage. "Some flower has finally unfolded and blossomed...the young man has received...a grounding that allows him to reconnect with some creativity [i.e., something feminine] that would have frightened him when he was younger...eventually, at fifty or fifty-five, we feel a golden ring on the finger again" (Bly, 1990, p.221). The challenge to men in the second half of life is to become an advocate for a young man's development, but especially at the time the young man is in Bly's sixth and seventh stages: the arrival of the mentor and the apprenticeship. Maturity, a basis of elderhood, is possible only after having reached a point where the elder is able to express a balance of both masculine and feminine energy. He must then utilize this balance of energy as a model for the next generation.

ELDER

Arrien

Anthropologist Angeles Arrien also believes there are eight stages of development. She derives her model from her review of cultures throughout the world. In exploring some myth she comes up with eight "gates" through which we must pass if we are to fully mature.

<u>Arriens Stages</u> (Elderhood in **bold**)
Youth

1. The silver gate	Challenge: birth and all that is new.
2. The white picket fence	Challenge: taking a look at the roles we play.
3. The clay gate	Challenge: looking into the mystery of sensuality and sexuality.

Middle Age

4. The black and white gate	Challenge: facing our fear and pride.
5. The rustic gate	Challenge: reviewing our creativity and assessing whether it aligns with our life calling and passions.

Maturity

6. The bone gate	Challenge: **reclamation of the authentic self so as to allow modeling of character and integrity.**
7. The natural gate	Challenge: **reviewing the contentment of our past life and what brings contentment now.**
8. The gold gate	Challenge: **letting go of attachments and embodying spiritual work which includes managing fear.**

Arrien's description of the stages of life is almost too abstruse for me. She does offer, however, another view of the challenge of elderhood. She teaches that the goal of the first part of life is to "seek success" and that this requires exploring our strengths and talents. The challenge of the first two gates and the white picket fence passage is in this exploration. In the middle of life she believes we transform and begin to reclaim our authentic selves, selves that were confused and masked by our exploration of roles and opportunities for success and our response to social expectations.

Her study of multiple cultures leads Arrien to suggest that the challenge of late life is to develop your character. Also, she asserts this requires being generative, compassionate and wise. This character development leads to mentoring, coaching and stewardship of people. In her model, the first elder quality is the challenge at the bone gate — reclamation of the authentic self to allow modeling of character and integrity. An example of this type of modeling is living the life of the blessing *way:* committing daily to setting sacred intention through prayer or some type of visible ceremony, giving gratitude and making a life affirming action at least once daily (Arrien, 1998)

Moore and Gillette

I reviewed in Chapter III the four archetypes of Sovereign, Lover, Warrior and Magician. Much of the material there came from the work of Robert Moore, a psychoanalyst, and his co-author, Douglas Gillette, a mythologist and counselor. These men found a consistent pattern throughout world cultures in male growth and development. They refer to their seven stages as stages of initiation. They found that masculine initiation in most cultures was a process with numerous steps.

<u>Moore and Gillette's Stages</u> (Elderhood in **bold**)
Youth

First stage of initiation	Challenge: a man becomes a Quester for something he lacks but senses it as his mission.
Second stage of initiation	Challenge: locating the qualities in himself he longs to have, he begins by seeing them only in other persons, objects and institutions.
Third stage of initiation	Challenge: experiencing the power of King, Lover, Warrior, and/or Magician energy in oneself.

Middle Life

Fourth stage	Challenge: where at first the man only had a slight grasp of his mission (and then was almost possessed by it), here he realizes the work necessary to develop into maturity.

Maturity
Fifth stage   Challenge: **mastering of the power** (i.e. King, Lover, Warrior or Magician)
Sixth stage of initiation   Challenge: **steward one's powers for the sake of others thus bringing our capacities into service.**

The last stage is where, as we mature we move from "possession" of skill and wisdom to "use" these resources for the sake of people and Earth. There are millions of men who have reached fifth degree initiations who are competent but they "have not yet begun to see that their remaining and most critical challenge is one of stewardship for the community of Earth" (Moore, 1993b, p.202). Being grown up means that we utilize our wisdom for the sake of others. Our North American focus on second-half-of-life as recreation and retirement can limit us to a fifth-degree initiation at best.

The first of three ways to move into elder status in my opinion, then, is to decide whether moving into elderhood is necessary to complete human development. Erikson told us that adulthood is defined in part as facing the crisis of generativity versus the despair of believing we have nothing to offer. Erikson's final crisis is to avoid despair about our mortality through a four-fold balance he calls ego integrity.

The poet, Robert Bly, takes us in a different direction. Bly asserts that growing up requires an apprenticeship to adulthood. After completing the training satisfactorily in the apprenticeship, we let go of many of the tools of growing up. We become self-actualized, fulfilling our potentials and setting our own standards. Bly says that we accomplish this through a balanced expression of both masculine and feminine energy. This is another way of reaching Erikson's ego integrity.

Arrien says that one goal in maturity is to let go of attachments and social expectations and incorporate our spiritual work. We could call this "following our heart". She lays out the challenge that older people are responsible for modeling integrity and good character. Older people who want to express elder qualities agree with her.

Moore and Gillette put development into the framework of initiations. The final challenge in their seventh stage of initiation is for us to steward our elder power, our wisdom, for the sake of others. They add to the previous three stage theories the step where we demonstrate for others that we have been initiated into adulthood.

It is possible to reach full maturity and avoid the developmental stage of elderhood. We can live a rich life; have fun and model many adult attributes without becoming an elder. However, an elder is a spiritual person whose maturity includes a passion for being a celebrant, saving Earth, mentoring the young and passing on a legacy in the form of story. Why concern ourselves with becoming an elder, though, when we feel we have already contributed a lot as a parent, a spouse, a citizen and a worker? Both the elder and the community must experience the energy of elderhood before either can have the peak experience of being fully alive, flourish and thrive. All adults are sixth-level initiates, but the elder has balanced in a fourfold way, has reclaimed their authentic self and has become a model of good character and ego integrity.

The Initiation of an Elder

Unlike for a youngster, the elder's journey is not one of becoming a unique psychological individual. The elder, having spent decades defining self, moves toward being initiated into a journey of partnership and community. This shift occurs in midlife and is so important that it usually disrupts the person's peace. There can be feelings of boredom, disillusionment with life, the disappearance of the dream we created in our youth. There is some regret and a heightened sense of our mortality and life's limited duration. A ceremony or initiation rite that facilitates the transition from midlife into elderhood can mitigate the difficulty of the transition into life's final stage.

The rituals of initiation and rites of passage function to move individuals through transition periods in their lives. They can have the effect of making the transition transformative. They give transitions personal and cultural significance. In the West, we have practices that are common to transitions, like a Mexican-American family honoring their daughter's transition into adulthood in the *Quincinera*. Or in the gold watch dinners where we define older people as "retired" when they turn age 65. These practices are common to our experience and imply that we are in the midst of transitions, but some lack the solemnity a ritual of initiation. Many cultures have initiation ceremonies for children who have become capable of sexual reproduction. To some, the word "initiation" means "puberty rites by virtue of which adolescents gain access to the sacred, to knowledge, and to sexuality by which, in short, they become human beings" (Eliade, 1958, p.132). However, a person can also be initiated into a fraternity, a marriage or the priesthood. We have learned much about initiation from the puberty rites of various cultures. There are many life transitions that rituals can facilitate.

The preparation and the testing of the initiates in most rites of passage are commonly the responsibility of the elders. The supervision of initiations by older people is needed but it makes sense only if these people have been initiated themselves or, through some other process, have taken ownership of their elderhood. Westerners have a grasp of some of the psychological functions of rites of passage, but this is the extent of elder knowledge about transitions in most cultures of the New World. I believe that the four aspects of transition as the West views and values them are shock, resistance, exploration and adaptation. Parents, grandparents and other mentors must understand that the process of change has these four challenges, but there is a spiritual mystery about growth and development that we need to respect as well. There is also the personal, unique dimension of growth as well.

Sacred Elderhood

My belief is that we need to integrate the sacred mystery with the psychological and social purposes of celebrating an individual's life transitions. We can find a microcosm of our more complex secular civilization in small, more primitive societies, past and present that were more in touch with the sacred mysteries. What we call primitive is what we once were! As society evolves, people become different and more advanced technologically than their predecessors. Modern people live longer, know more about the science of things, and are more complex intellectually. This *advancement* has its limitations. In primitive, less complex cultures people are more aware of their relationship to the Universe and are almost unable to separate the sacred from the secular. Aspects of the holy enter most phases of their life. Being born, reaching puberty and even visiting another culture are all acts that fall within the sacred sphere among many indigenous people. These are transitions, and all transitions mean that a form of birth and death is experienced. The "shock" and "resistance" we respect in the West are reactions to both a new challenge (a birth) and the close of something familiar (death).

Modern, advanced cultures have lost confidence in many sacred practices like prayer and rites of passage. To us they seem speculative, amorphous and a waste of time. As cultures evolve, the challenge of change becomes greater, the pace picks up and time management becomes essential. In managing time and coping with change — hallmarks of the modern stress manager — we are inclined to discard the least concrete and least useful from our behaviors. We believe that sacred practices only work if we have faith in them. However, "as we move downward on the scale of civilizations...we cannot fail to note an ever increasing domination of the secular by the sacred" (Van Gennep, 1960, p.2). In the world of primitive people, a people usually can't pass from one sacred level to the next without going through some kind of ritual.

In the secular world of the West, a person passes from midlife into the second half of life by intellectual and economic means. Our churches have the word elder in their parlance, but today, even religion gives much less sacred meaning to the role than did the sacred institutions of ancient times. We identify those who have passed into the second half of life by looking to secular institutions such as the Social Security Administration, the workplace, and the American Association of Retired Persons. These organizations define when we are "old enough" or "too old". Each of these groups honors our old age economically through stipends and price breaks. These institutions do have the effect of moving us into adulthood. However, an initiation ritual could attribute a divinely sanctioned meaning to a person's passage into old age. Ritual places people within the context of the culture's myths and traditions, giving them recognition and confirmation that a transition has occurred.

Our fear of aging has contributed to our fear of old people. The mode today is to dismiss most old traditions as suffocating, slow and unproductive. In pre-industrial times, the elders, utilizing ritual to imprint on our brains, passed on values and attitudes without many questions from generation to generation. However, we have more confidence today in the resilient young than the wise old. Our emphasis is on rebellion against the traditions of the fathers and solidarity within our peer group. With the influence of 21st century initiated elders the young might develop trust more easily.

Phases of Initiation

With an eye toward facilitating the development of mature people then, I will define the elements of an initiation ceremony that honors the elder rite of passage. Most rites of passage, from those of indigenous cultures to the early Christian rituals to the process of incorporating a recruit into the military, have three phases. These phases in order are: separation, threshold and incorporation (Van Gennep, p.11).

Separation comprises behaviors that suggest the detachment of a person from an old set of cultural conditions. It is the first of the three phases. All transitions have both losses and gains. Something ends while, at the same time, new opportunities present themselves. The separation phase of rites is like a small death. In indigenous cultures, initiates are sometimes buried or required to lie motionless during the separation phase of a rite. Some initiates are forced to live for a time with masked men who symbolize the dead. For military recruits the focus is on accepting a number and a uniform. Then they face the dreaded military haircut which "cuts away" old images of self and begins to define the soldier as a member of a new community. Cutting hair is common to many ancient rites of passage. This act connotes a dedication of a part of ourselves to the new condition of life we enter while relinquishing the part we leave behind.

During the next phase, the threshold phase, the state of mind of the initiate and her status in her community is uncertain. This is common to all of us when we pass through important life transitions. We lose balance and drift between the "devil and the deep blue sea". This threshold phase is like land that has been plowed but not yet seeded. The initiate encounters their limits and steps formally into the unknown. This requires training and mentoring because the initiate is lost, homeless and usually confused. In some social organizations, this is the time of instruction that precedes confirmation as a member. The instruction is usually secret and imparts knowledge allowed only among initiates who are passing through the threshold phase. Those cultures and institutions that have utilized rites of passage for centuries believe the new knowledge imprints the initiate, as a seal impresses wax, with the characteristics of a new state of being.

In the last phase, the incorporation phase, the initiates are enfolded by a community that recognizes them as new members whose initiation is complete. Among the Zuni of New Mexico, men wearing masks during the threshold phase removed their masks during incorporation, the last part of the initiation ritual. By this act they show the initiate that they really are men, not gods as they pretended earlier, and want him to join them as an equal (Bunzel, 1932, pp.516-517). In the military, the recruits are awarded their stripes as symbols of their incorporation into the ranks of fully trained soldiers. In this third phase, the initiate's passage is consummated. They are stable once again and, therefore, have rights and obligations to the community and are expected to follow customs and ascribe to delineated ethical standards.

Initiation Process
Introduction

The person who would be an initiate in this honoring of elderhood can expect the full process to take no less than six months. However, the decision about when the ritual reaches the threshold and incorporation phases belongs to the elder initiate. When the initiate feels they are ready to accept the mantle of elderhood, the initiation begins. It begins with the initiate's decision to participate in the rite and ends with a ceremony. I recommend assigning the role of ritual elder to another person who is in the second half of life whom the initiate trusts. Because we have not honored elders in this culture for so many generations, we may have a hard time identifying people we feel express elder energy. Rites of passage historically have been largely for men and supervised by men. As you search for elders to assist in this ritual, however, remain open to calling upon both men and women, young and old.

Consider the crone ceremonies that are increasingly visible today. They are intended to honor the wisdom of the older women and are rites of passage. Crone ceremonies are based on historical tradition where it was believed that "after menopause, menses were retained within as a source of power and magical purpose" (Reif, 2003, p.54). Women embracing the role of crone are accepting the mantle of elderhood. At the celebration during the incorporation phase, you will want to feel free to include all those people most important to you, male or female, child or adult.

You will want to tune each of the three phases to your own taste but below I have outlined a possible model for you to use. To begin a transition from adulthood into the highest level of maturity—"elderhood"— you need to let go of aspects of your sense of self and remain open to new ones. In the military the recruit is sent away from their community to boot camp where they are given a number and told to act like the others, to forget their normal routine and develop personal habits forced on them by the drill instructor. The modern Western elder accomplishes the separation, however, through gentler means including affirmation, prayer and symbolic ceremony.

Part I
Separation
Intent: To let go of aspects of self and open ourselves to others. The initiate would benefit from reflecting on these questions:
1. How might I shift my use of my time and resources to a service orientation?
2. In what ways can I address the issue of my own mortality?
3. Which of my life experiences have I framed negatively? Can I now reframe them with a positive view after grieving their passage?
4. Who have I not forgiven? How am I wasting energy on resenting people who let me down a long time ago?
5. How can I let loose my grip and "just be" without loosing control?
6. How do I know that I have wisdom?
7. Have I bought into the prejudice toward older people and do I believe my gray hair makes me useless?
8. In what way could I be a source of blessing to both people and Earth?
9. How can I integrate libido drives like maintaining physical beauty, obtaining power and position into *thanatos* drives like service, contemplation, conservation and mentoring?
10. What am I resisting about balance in a fourfold way? Is my greatest challenge in the spiritual, intellectual, physical or psychological realm?

The Players: Most of the time in this phase of initiation, the initiate will be alone. Gradually they will be encouraged to seek out other elders they feel express an elder nature.

Process: Enter the questions and your responses in a journal or diary. Journaling is an important element of your rite at all three stages. Journaling is a way of ritualizing the process of asking yourself the questions. Writing in a journal is a tried and true method of imprinting new concepts. However, you may also want to add symbolic actions that express your intentions and mark this time of separation from your old ways.

Other rituals the initiate could utilize include the burying or burning of paper on which has been written those aspects of your life you are letting go. Some initiates create an altar or add to an existing one some significant artifacts. In honoring the death that is separation, you and your ritual elder, or you alone, could go on a daylong hike. During this time you could consider the questions. On the day of the walk try fasting until after sunset. Fasting symbolizes a cleansing and helps us reach atonement, at-one-ment, with nature. As you walk, observe how nature reaches out to you with signs and symbols of your life purpose, inherent gifts, personal values and fears. Look at the evidence of passage in fallen trees, trampled flora and dying leaves. Find a natural item that symbolizes your separation and bring it home.

Part II
Threshold

Intent: The intent of the threshold phase in the elder initiation is to incubate the future. Answers to the questions above will coalesce to form a new foundation for a new mission as elder. The difference between the threshold period in most people's lives and the threshold of the elder initiation is the maturity of the person seeking this ritual. Threshold is a time of education and training for initiates in rites of passage. The person who is in the second half of life, however, has gathered much knowledge and has long life experience. Unlike the initiate who is joining a church as a young girl or a boy who is passing through puberty, the elder will do most of their threshold training alone.

The Players: Where, for example, the catechumen in the Catholic Church can depend on the priest to educate them during threshold, the elder must walk alone most of the time in their initiation. The catechumen, usually a neophyte Catholic, lacks the experience of the elder. Elders can learn from others, but the goal in the elder threshold rite is to tap the energy of the elder within. The other side of this issue is the difficulty in finding people who celebrate their elderhood. In the same way that I found people whom I called elders, I would challenge the elder initiate to identify within the community at least three people who meet the following criterion: A person who approaches being:

Seasoned, and is a source of life-giving energy
Knows their limitations and is skillful
Who has an unconquerable spirit
Who is knowledgeable, aware and filled with insight
Who is intuitive, passionate, spiritual and sensuous.

The three elders will play a role in the incorporation phase as well but during the threshold phase they can be an important resource. Bounce the questions off these people and enter a discussion with each about your responses. You will likely find the North American elder shy and resistant, but pursue them. Once they learn that they play a role in supporting your quest for elderhood, they will want to contribute something.

Another player is the ritual elder. During incorporation, the ritual elder will be your advocate and representative at the incorporation ceremony, but in the threshold phase engage with the ritual elder as you would a good brother or sister. Share your responses to the questions. Listen for their responses, as you will with the other three elders. The ritual elder's role in your rite is to facilitate the incorporation ceremony using the help of the other three. You will need to find a person who is comfortable with ritual and who is willing to facilitate. You might want to consider a teacher, a thespian or a minister.

The key player in the threshold phase, however, is the elder initiate. Utilizing the stepping-stones of wisdom, contemplation, listening, reflection and meditation, you will have to teach yourself how to become more elder like. You need, therefore, to create ground for use of these tools and, at the same time, create sacred space.

If the initiate went for a walk in nature they began forming sacred space. Let's turn now to the process of threshold. It is a sacred ceremony because the experience of it is utterly private, inexpressible and awesome. In this ceremony, the initiate is left alone with their perception of the Universe.

Process: The elder initiate will now go on retreat. The form of this getaway is up to the initiate. It should last at least three days and three nights. The retreat will be in a place and done in a way that is sacred to the initiate. Sacred space is holy ground. Holy ground is created when someone sees us, hears us, recognizes us and then admires and affirms us. Since the initiate will be alone, the only source of recognition and affirmation outside oneself will be their version of the universal force that organizes us all. The burden of creating sacred space in threshold, therefore, will be on the initiate engaging prayer, affirmation or tools such as the stepping-stones of wisdom. The retreat could be a driving trip where you never settle in a particular place but spend most of your time alone on the road and in motels or camping grounds. For others it will mean traveling to a retreat center that invites people to stay for the purpose of contemplation and study. Others may want to leave people all together camping in the wilderness.

The elder will need to judge what role trial, challenge or risk will play in his ritual. Fasting again is recommended and is a trial for most, because the vessel cannot be filled until it is emptied. The threshold phase is a time of building new vision that fills the initiate. Journaling will nearly always enrich the process of transition. For some it is a challenge to put into words the things felt during initiation.

The threshold phase ends when the elder initiate believes they have given sufficient time to the process of transition. To some degree this is artificial because the exact moment a person completes a life change cannot be pinpointed. In three days and nights, the elder will have given themselves a good opportunity to contemplate the change, their past condition and their plans for the future. The final act in the threshold phase is to begin a return to the community. It is time to assess how an elder can act on their responsibility as an advocate for community. This is a good time to utilize the listening support of the ritual elder. The time away will have stirred things in the initiate. He/she may want to share one of the revelations they had on their time away. One way a person becomes personally linked with others is by opening up and sharing revelations. The last phase of this initiation involves reincorporation into the community. Any steps the initiate can take that begin the process of melding with their circle of friends and relatives are worth experimenting with as the day of the incorporation ceremony approaches.

Reflections On Threshold Phase

Once completing this phase, the elder will have a stronger feeling about what they want to do in the second half of life. This will, in turn, help them cope with the loss of what aspects of self they have had to sacrifice. During the threshold phase aimless wandering should begin to become a more purposeful exploration of the responsibilities and potentials of elderhood. The possibilities of elder expression will overshadow the traditional older person's response of retirement which often makes them less accessible to society.

Most ancient threshold rites of passage involved some hardship, risk or trial. The trial could have been psychological or spiritual in nature. The initiate who would join a Christian church must repent "sins" they previously perceived to be nothing but "errors". They must declare that they are ready to shift from an involvement with self to a more focused relationship with God. Symbolically, the catechumen cannot enter that part of the church building where communion or baptism takes place until they finish the incorporation phase and are "confirmed". In some countries the catechumen faces rites of exorcism during threshold. Threshold can take many years in older tribal cultures such as those in Africa.

The military recruit endures a series of ordeals during their threshold phase. These include trials of strength, sleeplessness, inspections, obstacle courses, battle practice, combat, and forced marches. Some cultures subject their initiates to tortuous rituals. In the Gulf of Guinea in the Congo of 1900, initiates into adulthood had their bodies mutilated and painted. Elders directed them to wander around in the forest naked and out of sight because during this part of their ritual they were presumed dead.

Other terms for threshold in history have been *marge*, the French word for margin, and the Latin, *liminal*, which means, "limit". In this phase the quester encounters her margin or limit of former self and steps beyond.

Becoming An Elder

Indigenous people experience threshold not only as a time to move from one stage of life to another, but they also attribute to it a divinely sanctioned meaning. A person's life is enriched by relating themselves personally to the myths and spirits of their tribe. Trial for them, therefore, increases the awareness of human frailty and encourages surrender to the universal force of which both people and nature are an integral dimension. Those who utilize the initiation called the vision quest, a rite similar to those practiced by Native Americans, spend at least three to four days in a wilderness place and make use of Native American artifacts and ritual believed to enhance the spiritual experience. The vision questers often report that they have experienced a "'deathwarding birth contraction' during the quest. When they rejoin their community they have a clearer understanding of themselves in relation to the natural environment, but also to the others to whom they return" (Foster, 1992, pp.21-25).

Part III
Incorporation

Intent: The goal of this final phase is to incorporate the initiate as an elder through a celebration built on an endorsement from the people in the elder's community. The initiate was a member of the community prior to their initiation filling other roles including employer, brother, sister, parent, friend, teacher, spouse, neighbor or child. The ceremony of incorporation renews their membership in society now with the additional role of elder. The ceremony is usually an experience of renewal for the participants as well as the initiate. In this stage of their initiation, the aspiring church member is confirmed as an active member of the church. She is now given access to holy sacraments such as baptism and communion, a privilege reserved for confirmed members. During incorporation, the military recruit is presented with clothing that makes them look the same as other members of the military — hence the name, uniform. They are given training that allows them to have an occupation. This allows them to play a specific role and in and on behalf of the military community they have joined.

Players: At minimum, five persons are needed in the ceremony. In addition to the elder initiate, the ritual elder will be present to act as facilitator. The community will be standing in a large square during the ceremony. On each of the four sides a spokesperson will be asked to represent the community. If the initiates were able to identify a few elder men and women during the threshold phase, they may want to call on them as spokespersons.

For the four spokesperson's roles, the initiates will want people whom they trust, who appreciate them and who are willing to step forward. This could include the initiate's children and spouse.

Process: The initiates have some things to do in preparation for the incorporation celebration. They will need to identify the players and confirm their willingness to act as spokespersons. They will then prepare a statement explaining what aspect of the self they will leave behind and what new characteristic they will adopt. Symbolically, threshold is a time of death — death of old ways of being. Incorporation is an opportunity to announce what it means to accept new ways — ways of elder expression. The initiate may want someone in his or her community to create a mantle. This could be a badge, a cloth wrap that hangs around the neck or even a garment. The ritual elder can advise the artist on the design. By accepting the mantle, the elder initiate symbolically accepts the responsibility and blessing power of elderhood. Finally, the initiate will define a method or ritual that will invoke the powers that are beyond them. They could identify God or spirits meaningful to them, or people of their community, as their sacred energy source.

While in the midst of the ritual, the initiate can experience a kind of rapture. The way they experience it will vary depending on their religious and social heritage. A brief statement or set of behaviors by the ritual elder can invoke the sacred but either the initiate or the ritual elder can assume this responsibility.

On the day of the ceremony, all persons will stand on the outside of the square, the sides of which will be defined by the presence of the spokespersons. The ritual elder will walk the initiate to the center of the square, where the initiate will remain. The square has historically symbolized stability and an established foundation. The four sides will represent the balance of the fourfold way: psychological, physical, spiritual and intellectual. They will also represent the four archetypes of Sovereign, Lover, Warrior and Magician. They will represent the four callings of elderhood: celebrant, mentor, wisdomkeeper and earthkeeper. Finally, the four sides will correspond to the four directions.

Structuring the gathering around the four directions of the compass as seen in the Judeo-Christian cross, the Hindu mandala and the even the Aztec Swastika calendar wheel, creates a whole, a balanced, symbolic representation of the self in harmonious relationship to creation. The four directions also represent the four seasons, the four quadrants of the heavens and the four dimensions.

The spokesperson for the Lover energy will stand in the Eastern direction. The East represents youthfulness, playfulness and spirituality in many spiritual traditions. The East also symbolizes the elder's role as one who blesses: celebrant.

In the South, the spokesperson will stand for Warrior energy such as assertiveness, and a commitment to high values that guides the elder as an advocate for people and the earth: earthkeeper.

In the West the spokesperson will remind the elder that he/she who expresses Magician energy is a teacher and is in service: wisdomkeeper.

The North side represents Sovereign energy: the mentor. The spokesperson the North announces that the community looks to the elder to be joyful in celebration of life and that they are responsible for utilizing their long life experience on behalf of younger generations. Each spokesperson will present one question for the elder initiate to answer spontaneously. The question is intended to provoke the initiate to consider each of the four elder roles.

As the end of the ceremony approaches, the initiate will be asked to speak. It is at this time that they will share a prepared statement about the meaning of the initiation to them. Also, they will have brought items discovered during the separation and threshold phases. These might include natural things such as stones or leaves. A walking stick may have been utilized during the walk.

The initiate must now, in some way, burn, bury or discard symbols that represent the past. Following this act of release, the ritual elder will bring forward the mantle of elderhood and present it to the initiate. The ritual elder will offer a blessing on behalf of the community and then request the persons gathered to approach, offering touch, blessings or some other demonstrative form of endorsement that shows their pleasure with the incorporation of this elder.

The process of incorporating the initiate into the community is the responsibility of the elder's friends and relatives. Therefore, their presence at the ceremony is essential. Hopefully, a number of these people have passed through their own threshold phases. Everyone present will understand to some degree the importance of the ceremony, even if they have not been oriented to the idea of an elder initiation. The gathered throngs are "birth attendants, midwives" (Foster, 1984, p.53). The role of community will become even more important as we look at the work a person must do to grow into elderhood.

Reflections On the Incorporation Phase

The subject of sacredness deserves further comment. In Arnold Van Gennep's review of worldwide rites of passage, he found that initiates were not in their usual earthly state during the high points of the rites. The rituals possessed elements of intense sacredness because of the emotions and images they stirred in both the initiate and the people participating in the ritual. For each initiate the meaning of sacred will differ. It usually is described as holy, religious, spiritual or divine. Invoking the influence of the sacred will usually be important to the person participating in the elder initiation, but each is free to judge this for themselves. A person who does not consider himself spiritual can accomplish something comparable by invoking the love and appreciation of their gathered friends and relatives.

Growing into Elderhood

Growing into elderhood is the third way an older person can embrace the role of elder as a way of being. The reader will recall the first was embracing elderhood as a stage of personal development. The second was subjecting oneself to an initiation process. Growing into elderhood probably will not happen just because we have lived a long life. The growth that is measured by reaching each stage of development is fourfold in nature, but my emphasis here is on psychological, intellectual and spiritual growth. We can mature and flower beyond our present state by choosing to grow in self awareness. Once we make this choice, we need to change attitudes, challenge biases and learn more. We will need to evaluate our values. Our behaviors will, as a result, become different.

In what you have read so far, there are a number of hints about where we could focus our commitment to growth into elderhood. I have asserted, for example, the importance of becoming balanced in a fourfold way. Carrying the mantle of elderhood will be easier if we first solve our psychological problems, seek to become centered spiritually, keep better care of our physical health and study philosophical writers such as those quoted throughout this book. Elders express a compatible and balanced energy from each of the four archetypes of elder expression mentioned above: Sovereign, Magician, Lover and Warrior. This facilitates a positive expression of the three personal roles of protector, provider and teacher that was referred to an earlier chapter. The full expression of masculine and feminine energy is another challenge. You will recall that Robert Bly asserts that the integration of these two energies is the last stage, the most mature stage, of personal development. An elder can also grow by committing to a review of the following attitudes, biases and expressions of values.

Myths About Aging

Our elder growth requires that we stop clinging to our myths about aging. This includes confronting the retirement myth mentioned earlier. Older people don't need less sleep than younger people but this is one of our myths. Older men and women don't become sexless. People who don't follow the bias of maintaining young beauty as long as possible appreciate elder beauty. Older people don't forget everything. "Of the 30 million Americans over the age of 65, only 10% show any significant loss of memory" (Dychtwald, 1990, p.38). One of my most ambivalent experiences is eating in a restaurant that has a special menu for older people. It is nice that the price is lower but the portions are also smaller. Who says old people eat less than young people? Could it be that American restaurateurs have an image of elders as so frail that they get tired half way through a normal sized meal?

The developmental task here is to overcome our inclination to let go of the child within as we age. The wise elder retains his connection to youthful vitality. She balances libido and *thanatos* energy. Saint Augustine said, "Let your old age be childlike, and your childhood like old age; that is, so that neither may your wisdom be with pride, nor your humility without wisdom" (Augustine, 1945) At each stage of life there is within us a coexisting presence of the child and the elder, the archetypal images of youth and age. Our negative images of aging result in large part from our denial that we retain libidinal drives, the youthful, spontaneous and resilient drives that continually bring adventure to life.

Accessibility

Elders need to be available. The problem with the retirement myth is that many of us focus our energy after our mid-life work career ends on being left alone and out-of-touch. Because we have built a tradition of less visibility, older people assume their presence is unnecessary. They travel more or actually move away from their extended family thus reinforcing the myth that elders are less useful. Genuine wisdom is attributed to those with the "capacity to 'feel', to exhibit 'compassion' and 'generosity' toward others, and to develop intimate, insightful and empathetic relationships" (Suzuki, 1992, p.225). Building relationships requires regular exposure to those with whom we relate. Eldering is more an experience in being and less in doing. Elders needn't do anything while remaining within reach, but they must remain within reach.

If our focus was on accessibility, retirement would look more like harvesting, accepting our role as mentors, being sources of blessing, backing up the struggling nuclear family, and caring for Earth. Rabbi Schachter-Shalomi says that harvesting is a second half of life practice involving a celebration of the impact we have had in our lifetime. Harvesting then leads to a passion for leaving a legacy for the future.

Celebration

The second half of life can be a time of celebration! Old age could be the time when we reap what we have sown. How about redefining our increased recreation as *re-creating* through self-discovery, conservation of Earth or fostering the healthy growth of children! For me recreation is a big part of the second half of my life. If we have the financial resources and are blessed with adequate health we have every right to play as much as possible. Celebration of life includes being able to live with the consciousness of "social convention be damned!" Having lived a long life is plenty of reason to be more spontaneous, less organized and very playful.

> When I am an old woman I shall wear purple
> With a red had that doesn't go, and doesn't suit me
> And I shall spend my pension on brandy and summer gloves
> And satin sandals, and say we've no money for butter.
> I shall sit down on the pavement when I am tired
> And gobble up samples in shops and press alarm bells
> And run my stick along public railings
> And make up for the sobriety of my youth. (Joseph, 1991, p.1)

We can confuse, however, recreation with running away. If we embrace the prejudice toward older people we can easily get the impression that we are in the way, not needed and have little to contribute. Let's be fun loving and in the process make it more enjoyable for the community to want us around. A constructive form of retirement behavior is centering through contemplation of all that we have sown, while at the same time staying in town more often and getting out so others can get a piece of us!

Second half of life celebration could begin with a review of our life. When we reach 60 years of age, we can look back and see most of our life cycles. To have traveled through each stage of development is quite an accomplishment. The errors and omissions for which we are responsible can be reframed as "opportunities for growth". This is part of what gerontologists call life review. "The life review is...a progressive return to consciousness of past experience, in particular the resurgence of unresolved conflicts which can now be surveyed and integrated" into our enhanced elder sense of self (Butler, 1974, p.534).

One of the most satisfying psychotherapeutic tools I have used in counseling is the task of reframing. This process requires a review of a portion of a person's life history that we find repugnant and reevaluating the events and look for hope and opportunity. Once discovering the doors that were opened for growth in each life experience, we can reframe the memory as a positive event. This literally allows us to reclaim energy previously devoted to calling past events negative or hurtful. Life review is more than recalling our past. We can heal the injury resulting from a trauma or a disappointing life experience. This reframing must include, however, room in our life for grief and loss. The pain of some losses never goes away but can become lessened. Grief is integral to life because loss is common to life.

Painful memories affect how we act in the present when we endeavor to avoid experiences in the present that look like the painful ones of our past. We are often drawn into circumstances that are similar because we unconsciously want to heal the injuries and let go of our regret. Through the use of the wisdom tools of contemplation and meditation, we can recall the old memories and reframe them because of our maturity and readiness for celebration.

Forgiveness

A key to the process of reframing is forgiveness. In the second half of life a person "must come to terms with his grievances and guilts—his view of himself as victim and as villain...." (Levinson, 1978, p.224). An older person must not only accept their shadow but also forgive those people whose shadow has victimized them. The elder is acquainted with her shadow but doesn't let it run her life. We can "acknowledge and assume responsibility for the damage we have incurred or caused. Working through [the resulting injury] calls for...healing forgiveness" (Bianchi, 1982, p.65). Rudyard Kipling wrote in this excerpt from his poem, "If":

> If neither foes nor loving friends can hurt you;
> If all men count with you, but none too much;
> If you can fill the unforgiving minute
> With sixty seconds' worth of distance run—
> Yours is the Earth and everything that's in it,
> And—which is more—you'll be a Man my son!

To not forgive is to invest present energy in things past. Holding a grudge is work that wastes present day resources. The person who let us down isn't even aware of how much work we put into remembering what we call "their unforgivable act." In my training with the Spiritual Eldering Institute (1997-98), we did an exercise called A Testimonial Dinner for My

Severe Teachers. The trainer asked us "What if you invited your lifelong enemies to an imaginary banquet?" In the spirit of reframing, then, we made a list of the guests we would invite. Next to each guest's name, we listed what he or she did that was difficult for us. Finally, next to each difficulty, we listed its benefit. We looked for the unexpected gift in the acts of the enemies on our list. Finally, we forced ourselves to write down something about the difficulty for which we are now grateful. In this exercise we did not have to forgive the guests. Forgiveness in this case was the name we gave to finally giving up the burden of anger or hurt, which had kept us in the role of victim (Iser, 1996, pp.52-53).

Forgiving is not just excusing. It is a way to save energy in the second half of life. For the wise elder forgiveness is an empathetic healing of memory. Wisdom allows elders to recognize their severe teachers as victims themselves. The elder enters into the pain that they have caused others through error, a misuse of power or uncontrolled anger. Through such empathy, a cleansing takes place. They then forgive hurt without harboring resentments and free themselves from the energy-consuming bitterness of holding a grudge.

Confronting Our Mortality

Mortality is about being a physical person, about physical reality including death. In my criticism of the paradigm of traditional aging that leads in too many cases to one becoming elderly, I do not mean to suggest a denial of physical depletion. However, our preoccupation with depletion concerns me. I rode Amtrak between Portland, Oregon and Tucson, Arizona a few years ago. A man of my father's generation and I struck up a stimulating conversation about family, work and other things meaningful to both of us. Another man sat down at our table a short time later. He was also of my new friend's generation. Very soon the two men began an endless conversation about the physical ailments they had experienced. Their engrossment with their experience of depletion overwhelmed and replaced our earlier discussion. In a way, each man made himself inaccessible to me by dwelling on his fear of mortality.

For men in particular, the challenge of confronting mortality is to convert our life long commitment to "kill and survive" to an attitude of "die and become" (Bianchi, 1982, p.181). German poet and novelist Johann Goethe wrote:

> Die and Become.
> Till thou hast learned this
> Thou are but a dull guest
> On this dark planet.

Depletion is real yet gradual. If we tap the rhythm of elderhood, it influences us to slow down and listen to deeper impulses and question the hectic pace of youth. In Mitch Albom's, *Tuesdays With Morrie*, the terminally ill older man, Morrie, says to his interviewer, "Well, the truth is, if you really listen to that bird on your shoulder—*if you accept that you can die at any time*—then you might not be as ambitious as you are...The things you spend so much time on—all this work you do—might not seem as important. You might have to make room for some spiritual things" (Albom, 1997, pp.83-84).

Morrie utilized his impending death as a teaching tool. By reflecting deeply on our impermanence, we can be energized in the present because we accept that we must deal with the contingency of time. Morrie's acceptance of his mortality helped move him toward elderhood. He energized himself to share his wisdom, now! People who have had near-death experiences often have a reduced fear of and deeper acceptance of mortality. It is common for them to have an increased interest in service and an enhanced grasp of the importance of love, community and accessibility. They lose some interest in materialistic objectives because "you can't take it with you."

The specter of death can beckon us to move into the elder stages of personal development. If older persons don't face depletion and death directly, they find themselves in a trap resisting the flow of time. In my spiritual eldering work, we call this, "the box of unlived life." On one side of the box is the future. To move into the future, we must accept our mortality. Most of us fear this reality, however, causing us to look away and to look back into the past. The past is on the other side of the box. If we haven't reframed our failures and disappointments, we won't want to face them. We are then forced to live within the box, without the ability to look toward the future and view our past with poise and confidence (Iser, 1996, p.5).

Though I believe that death will be one of the most powerful experiences in my life, Western culture works hard to help me deny my imminent death. Media and advertising try to cultivate a belief in immortality, because this is what we are interested in buying. Most human fear is rooted in our fear of death. Life can scare us because of its unpredictability. In my quest for elderhood, I keep considering death, dying and mortality. This consideration is at least more productive than an outright denial of my death, but I still have a long way to go in accepting the rhythm of death in our lives. It is important to confront our mortality if we believe in both the spiritual realm and in the task of conserving energy in the second half of life. My spirituality includes the belief that life is eternal through the medium of the soul. Embracing mortality leads to energy conservation because we end up investing less time in the fear of things over which we have little control.

Developing Confidence in Your Wisdom

I made reference above to the energy of the elder within in the psyche of an older person. Once we access this energy actively, we can be more elder like. My description of an elder may feel more like an aspiration than a real possibility, but there is within each "elder potential". The Spiritual Eldering Institute has conceptualized the elder within as your 120 year-old selves. In the Bible 120 years is a symbolic "age of wisdom". The elder within is the archetype of our fully realized self who has done life review and forgiveness work, who has let go of biases about aging, faced mortality and integrated libido and *thanatos* energy. The elder within is a source of hope that one can become an elder.

As a person seeking a fuller expression of elderhood, you will need to contact your inner source of wisdom and receive occasional guidance. This is your elder within who resides in your heart and exists beyond time and space. You can visit with your ancient, fully actualized self and obtain reassurance whenever you need it. Your elder within can guide you with knowledge of your future. Try this exercise taught to me by the Spiritual Eldering Institute. In this guided meditation you can make an appointment to visit your elder within at any time. To begin this exercise, find a quiet place to sit.

The Meditation

Record the following on audiotape so that you can play it back to guide yourself through the imagery. Become aware of your breathing. Don't change its rhythm. Become more aware of your in-breath and your out-breath. Now, begin counting from your current age up to 120. As you count, picture yourself walking up a flight of stairs that lead to a door. Once reaching the door, knock on it and enter. Your evolved spiritual self, your elder within or inner crone greets you with a warm hug. Gaze into the eyes and experience unconditional love and reassurance about your progress in life. Ask your elder within for guidance about a specific concern with which you have been grappling. After asking, quietly remain receptive to the response and allow it to imprint itself on your consciousness [Turn off the tape recorder for a while].

When you receive your answer, turn on the recorder once again. Look once more into the eyes of this inner grandparent and hear these parting words, "Journey on with confidence and with blessings as you proceed on your path. Visit me again whenever you need further guidance." Bid him or her goodbye, turn and walk through the door, down the steps slowly and return to your point of departure — your present chronological age.

Sit quietly for a few moments. Open your eyes when you are ready. Turn off the recorder. You can now return regularly to visit your inner elder and be reassured of your gifts and wisdom.

End of Meditation

To develop confidence in your wisdom, first ask yourself, "Am I wise?" Your answer will be impacted by your confidence in long life experience. There are wise young people but it usually takes decades to develop wisdom. The wise person is paradoxically willing to share their insight while at the same time waiting for the right time to do so. Wisdom is insight and intuition synthesized through love and hope. We contain our fears and shyness about speaking our mind when sharing wisdom. The wise person is more concerned with being accessible than being verbal, however. If I remain inaccessible and quiet, for fear that my long life experience has yielded little wisdom, maybe I will waste something needed by others.

Second, make lists of all your roles: parent; worker; community leader; voter; hobbyist; friend; spouse; entrepreneur; traveler; pet owner; etc. Then list next to each role how many years you have been playing each. Now add up the years. This extensive experience could benefit others if shared. The task of experimenting with and provoking social change, and developing new ideas and tools is assigned to the young. How efficiently can they progress without the wisdom of the elders?

Finally, don't fear that your interference will cause a repetition of old ways and discourage creativity. We "have to enlist the elders, who have traditionally been the wardens of culture, to help and guide us in the vital process of reversing deculturation and of crafting the new myths on which reculturation can be based" (Gutmann, 1994, p.253). The young are vigorous and will not allow a return to ways and methods no longer useful, but they lack the memory of simpler days, less violence and a greener Earth. The elder of today remembers when families were more functional, when no freeways existed, when we could cut down a Christmas tree near our home. The elder remembers when childcare was not an industry but rather an occasional need, when fathers stayed with their families and women didn't have babies out of wedlock. We may not return to those experiences, but the memory of them influences the elder.

Loosening Our Grip

Growing into elderhood is spiritual work. Spiritual work involves seeking the meaning of existence or learning to accept aspects of it as mystery. The elder is a seeker and is thus on a spiritual journey that "grows him up". The key to spiritual work is 'letting go and letting God" as highlighted in the *Via Negativa* path. This requires letting go our grip on our ego, that aspect of self that is not immortal. The spirit is immortal. Once letting go our egos, we need then to come to the understanding that we are a servant of a higher purpose than self. Once letting go of our grip on our egos, we are left with a bit of a void that enables a discovering of that higher purpose and helps us fill it. The loosening of our grip can cause some movement away from individualism and toward union with the community and nature. In our youth we feed our ego. In elderhood we honor our ego but experience ourselves as one of many egos in an interrelated human community. A synergy occurs between elders and community that energizes both.

The concept of loosening our grip is considerably different than "losing your grip"! Our hands' grip may diminish as well as we age, but this is also quite different than loosening our grip. There is no reason for a healthy older person to diminish intellectually or psychologically. In fact, the ability to loosen our grip is proof of increased intellectual and psychological growth. The balanced elder is a good "stress manager". Effective stress managers understand above all else how much they can handle. Concerning what they can't handle, they loosen their grip a bit. This allows them to use their given pool of energy for just those challenges within their energy range.

To loosen your grip interpersonally means, for example, to take criticism lightly. The elder knows that criticism is discriminating judgment, not condemnation. To loosen your grip psychologically means, in part, to loosen up about fears by letting them pass on through you. Fears take a toll when you hold onto them, letting them take you out of your center, your spirit. To loosen your grip philosophically, stop asking why and follow your heart with confidence in your wisdom, your intuition and your ability to recover from occasional clumsy spontaneous acts. To loosen your grip in parenting is to stay within reach of your adult children but to get "out of their face". They need your presence, but not your instruction.

She of the loosened grip, while not losing control, is more relaxed. Being relaxed brings about qualities like patience, clearer perception, an awareness of the present and a desire to listen and talk less. He of the loosened grip is discerning. Discernment is an awareness of the divine in all. To be discerning is to discover the sacred in other people and creation as well. This is one of the most valuable qualities among mystics. Mystics are "keen on the *experience* of the Divine and will not settle for theory alone or *knowing about* the Divine" (Fox, 1983b, p.48). When we sit with an elder who is discerning, we will find them deeply attentive to us. Because they have let go their tight hold on many lesser things, they gather additional energy they can use to be open, patient and permeable to all you are saying. The discerning elder follows their intuition about what to do with what they have perceived in us. The discerning elder can not only put themselves out of the way so they can hear us, but they can also help us develop and trust in our own powers of discernment. This virtue "is a sort of sanctified common sense...It sees the humorous side of exaggeration..." (France, 1996, P.48). We have to loosen our grip before we can see the humorous side of things.

Balancing Our Psychic Energies

Those influences that emanate from our psyche I call the energies, both conscious and unconscious, make up the human personality. In Chapter V, I discussed those energies that weigh heavily in determining maturity. They include: the four archetypes—Sovereign, Lover, Warrior and Magician; the masculine and feminine energies; shadow energy; and the energy from each of the three roles of protector, provider and teacher of cultural tradition. Growing into elderhood includes utilizing these psychic influences in a way that is balanced. A balance of expression of the four archetypes results in a mature manifestation of emotional health. A controlled expression of shadow energy, on the other hand, is the goal of the wise elder.

There are bright energies and shadow energies common to the psychic imprint, or inborn pattern of expression, for each archetype. The task in maturity is to draw upon each of the four and also to keep under control the destructive shadow energy of each. A person who expresses himself or herself utilizing bright Sovereign energy, for example, is generative and celebrates new life in a joyful way. The Sovereign's shadow side would move a person to be destructive in his or her fear of new life. It is from the dark side of this archetype that a man or woman expresses power-over and is willing to degrade others. Growing into elderhood, then, includes an attempt to express bright sovereign energy as much as possible.

Lover energy brings about a playful and sensuous approach to living. At best, the person expressing bright Lover energy is intuitive and spiritual. They are in touch with the oneness of all people and feel connected with all creation. Shadow Lovers lack personal boundaries, however, and disrespect those of others. It feels like a dance between the bright side and the shadow side of an archetype. In a healthy expression, Lover means connection. In an unhealthy expression, it means over-connection as we forget to respect other people's need for privacy.

Magician energy brings about the healer in us and stimulates the teacher in us. The Magician is the master of knowledge and this archetype's concrete view of the world can protect us from the emotional irrationality of the Shadow Lover. Each archetype can protect us from the shadow of the other three. The Shadow Magician is manipulative, slippery and illusive. It is known as the Trickster in mythical history. She can be dishonest and lets her fears determine her reactions to people.

The Warrior, on good days, is assertive in the quest to reach lofty goals that take him or her beyond selfishness. Warrior energy is good for us as it causes us to establish safe boundaries, thus protecting us from the manipulative shadow Magician or the tyranny of the shadow Sovereign. The shadow Warrior perpetrates violence and can be sadistic and cowardly. The uncontrolled anger of this archetype abuses others and is feared by other people. Modern men are more confused about this archetype than the other three. In the attempt to move beyond from patriarchy, many men have confused shadow Sovereign energy with the assertiveness that comes from Warrior energy. As we relaxed our exploitative, patriarchal ways, we accidentally laid down the Warrior sword that has been essential in the protection of humankind.

Balancing our masculine and feminine energies requires an honoring of both. The 21st Century elder respects that they have both feminine and masculine traits, while at the same time understanding that gender expression changed considerably in the 20th Century from what it was in earlier times. The 21st Century elder understands that while seeking power is a masculine trait, more women today express masculine power-seeking energy as well.

The person who is in the second half of life is more likely to be contemplative than when they were when younger. This receptivity is a feminine trait. The use of power has changed in the past few decades. Men used to be identified with political and economic power, women with emotional and sexual power. Now, increasing numbers of professional women and increasing numbers of child-rearing men have both changed our view of the expression of masculine and feminine energies. Some things also seem never to change about men and women. "The woman...is experienced...as the source and giver of life...whereas the male... is one who <u>gained</u> his powers...The mother is experienced as a power of nature and the father as the authority of the society..." (Campbell, 1972, p.36). Honoring the masculine and the feminine includes considering the question, "Aren't some expressions or gender roles hard-wired into the psyche of both men and women?" This is a question which the elder must ponder.

Growing into elderhood requires confronting our compulsions, weaknesses and addictions. These are dark side issues, our human challenge. We are not just holy spirits. We are embodied spirits on the human journey as well as humans on a spiritual journey. The dark side of humanity is what I introduced above as the shadow. This is that part of us of which we are not proud. The shadow energies expressed by each of the four archetypes must be contained to some degree. These are the aspects of the self that we need to monitor, for they influence us to express destructive compulsive and addictive behaviors. An elder learns that people project their shadow onto others in trying to pretend they have no dark side. Test this by considering what behaviors or personality characteristics you like least in other people. An objective explanation for why we don't like people acting in those ways is that we don't like watching the behavior of our shadow in others. What we disapprove of in others' behaviors we don't enjoy in ourselves. Otherwise, why would we be so invested in other people's ways of being?

The elder enters into a dance with his shadow. This dance allows the shadow some expression, but it doesn't take control. Shadow energies only become destructive when they are not honored. In the elder's dance with shadow, he or she absorbs the shadow's power and doesn't attempt to repress it. This absorption converts shadow energy into a vitality that is stimulating but still potentially risky. If absorbed, it is neither repressed nor expressed. Try to imagine manipulation, anger or compulsion expressed at a low level of energy. Absorbed shadow energy can be invigorating. Elders continue this dance throughout their life.

Finally, balancing our psychic energies includes the living out of 21st Century gender roles. I have narrowed the list down to three: protector, provider, and teacher of cultural tradition. To assist the aspiring elder in this balancing act, you will find in the next chapter a review of these roles in action. However, before I end this chapter I want to tell you about one elder activity that has worked for me. It is the Elder Council in Portland, Oregon.

Elder Council

The Elder Council has been meeting quarterly for three years since 2001 to embrace the elder archetype. I organized this body to create a container of wise people who could both respond personally to my elderhood concept and grow into eldership with me. All sixteen of us men and women, aged 50 to 80 years of age, of the Council look forward to each gathering in large part because it is a sacred container where each person can practice elder behavior.

The Council convenes its quarterly gathering at 9:30 AM and ends the day at 3:00 PM. There are three parts when we gather: Opening, Word and Closing. The goal of the Opening activity is to create a sacred circle in which the council members focus on spirituality. The Council is made up of people of numerous religious traditions including New Thought, Catholic, Episcopal and Jewish. All the members share a passion for being involved in a spiritual community. The Word part of the gathering is defined in part by the season. For example, in the summer the council meets in a forest setting and brings their blessings to the land. In one winter meeting the group met at a meeting house on the grounds of a facility operated by an order of Catholic sisters. The Word for that gathering was end of life planning, embracing mortality and engaging in life completion activities. The table or alter is created differently each time the council meets. The items the council members place on the table represent each person's way of symbolizing the Word for that day.

The agenda for the spring meetings are influenced by this season of new life. The energy of the council in the spring comes from musing about how to stay in touch with the child within us. The summer focus is about ripening. In the fall the exercises and discussion relate in some way to harvest and the harvesting of long life. Winter meetings are concerned with end of life planning and embracing our mortality.

Activities include telling life stories, discussion of the meaning of elder expression for each person, offering of blessings for someone, Earth or some movement, doing life completion work, confronting our biases toward aging and other "personal elder work". The basis for the meeting is what is called, *council*. To meet in council is to meet together as peers, confident that each participant is willing to share wisdom and vision. It means to meet together to consider what might be possible without competition, without the struggle for position, recognition or the last word. Council is a form of deliberation practiced historically by indigenous people including Native Americans and Buddhist cultures as well.

To meet in council implies meeting as men and women without title, rank or constituency. Council is a profound forum where each, in turn, speaks truthfully, from the heart and where each listens with unconditional regard and great attention to the speaker. When we gather in council as our form, each expects that no one comes with prepared statements. Further, no one challenges any one else's statement but, rather, makes "I" statements to enhance a point made by another. In council each person's personal story is acknowledged, valued and urgently requested for elders.

With the ancient model of elder as our guiding archetype each member of the circle is willing to admit grief, ignorance, despair and a willingness to learn. Each is naked and honest in his/her speech. Each offers their wisdom as a harvesting of their long life experience and growing connection to other people and Earth. Each allows themselves to be enlightened and transformed by the others. Council process continues until consensus has been reached if a discussion has ensued. The Elder Council is energized by the recognition of a transpersonal power that both supports the council by its light and expresses itself through each council member.

CHAPTER SEVEN

Action Elderhood

What then is "action elderhood"? Are "action" and "elder" contradictory? One thing for sure, elder action does not resemble the energetic and decisive "man of action" archetype that our culture celebrates.

Action elders move towards that which has inherent satisfaction. They have energizing qualities that are libidinal and generative qualities that are *thanatos* driven. Action elderhood behavior includes actions that are just plain fun, that empower others, that conserve nature and bless the young. Action elderhood also honors the more limited energy pool in the elder's aging body, makes good use of the elder's long life experience, leaves a legacy and tells the elder's story.

Being an action elder can require activity, but action eldering is also "useless" like a large weeping willow tree, the tallest mountain in the range or the Grand Canyon. These sources of inspiration do nothing, yet they are sources of awe-inspiring beauty. They are models of serenity and strength. In their size they dwarf and place in perspective our worries and fears. Action elderhood means, in part, spending useless time with others: time not to do but rather to just be. Time to be a good listener and time to ask others important questions like, "Is your life working out the way you hoped?" "How are you feeling?" "Would you like to just sit quietly with me?" This is the quality of being accessible. Those for whom we could become a resource may need nothing more than someone capable of giving them attention.

The "useless elder" and the action elder are often the same. The useless elder blesses by giving full attention. Let us recall the meaning of sacred space: holy ground created when people are seen, heard, recognized, admired and affirmed by another. How do we explain the magic that occurs between the attending grandmother and the enraptured granddaughter? The relationship between the child and her parents can be limited by the multiple demands of raising her. She has, at the same time, a need to form her personality, often achieved by contrasting herself with what she defines as her parents' deficiencies. As grandparent, however, I can be wonderfully useless and waste time with my grandchildren. I can see clearly because I am not over invested in how she develops. If we are quiet willow trees for our grandchildren, for friends or the clerk at the store, we need not fade away as we age because people will gather beneath our shade.

The 21st Century provider, who is a good example of mature expression, is one who endows, not just supplies. He accommodates, not simply furnishes. He contributes while he fills up, and he replenishes those he serves. Let us look now at action elderhood and the provider role together. The way the elder endows is by their accessibility.

Giving Attention, Being Accessible

One of my mentors once told me that older people, in trying to be accessible, often get so impatient to upload information by talking with younger people that they forget the secret of mentoring which is: don't try to be a mentor! "Once the word gets out that someone has good ears," he said, "young people will come. It's like fishing. If we yank at the first nibble, the fish gets off the hook." I experimented with this idea by first asking myself what is the simplest form of being accessible and giving attention at the same time. I decided that it could begin with strangers on the street. Daily, I set a sacred intention by lighting a candle on my altar at home. I affirm that during the day I will give gratitude for grace in my life and look for ways to affirm life. This is the process ancient elders call a daily experience in "the blessing way". Finding ways to affirm life is not easy, however, so I try to look for simple ways to do it. Giving attention to a stranger affirms life.

It would be easy if every day some person came up to me and asked for help. But it requires more work than that. We can drive the streets, for example, and often find someone with a flat tire, someone needing a handout or someone needing directions. Helping these people is an example of affirming life. So is weeding your garden or contributing money to a conservation cause. Just greeting strangers more often, emanating friendliness and a desire to be available is being accessible. The elder can be action oriented by greeting others first and offering the first smile to the other. In this way, we take on the responsibility for offering a blessing and making the day a little less difficult for others. The accessible elder may make the first step by creating a dialogue with someone who might benefit from elder wisdom.

Facilitating Community

Keep in mind that we are creating a new way of being in the role of provider. A soul nourishing way to provide for, to endow and to fill up others is to improve the community in which they live. Our existence begins with dependence on others, and then we become conscious of ourselves and then, as we mature, we blossom into being responsible members of a community either in the form of family, neighborhood, social group or workplace. From community experiences we become aware of other communities we belong to: city, state, country, world, and then, Universe. The elder can have an impact on our country and world by facilitating community. Remember we are talking about regular folks here, not extraordinary characters like Mother Theresa or Jesus. Look at what action elderhood's potential impact on the community could be. Start with your neighborhood or your apartment building.

Let's walk along and observe a spiritual elder in their community. They have surveyed the area looking for ways to affirm life by being accessible, generative, attentive, available, patient. The elder observes, for example, that neighbors all have their own lawnmowers, video cameras, bicycles and barbecues, and seldom think about sharing their use. It is unlikely, the elder muses, that any single neighbor knows the names of more than a few of his fellow neighbors. Nearly all of the neighbors use babysitters that they bring in from other neighborhoods.

ELDER

Arriving at the park on the corner, the elder comes upon a teenager playing basketball. What possibilities for building community lie in this situation? The elder catches the boy's eye and says,

"Hello, don't you live on Aaron Court?"

"Yea," he says a little shy.

"The Hewett's live there. They used to live on our street," says the elder.

"They have a house next to ours," the boy reports as he once again shoots the ball.

"They have a boy your age don't they?" asks the elder.

"No, the girl that lives there is my age," says the boy.

"I am Terry Jones. We live on Stonehaven Court," offers the older man.

"Hi," says the boy.

As he begins to walk away, the elder says, "I sure hope the rain doesn't disturb your play. Have a good day." The boy waves and smiles partly because an older man has noticed him. The neighbors that the boy runs across usually say little more than "Hi". This was a simple yet different experience in building community facilitated by the older man. What might happen the next time the boy and the elder meet? The boy found the older man approachable and interested in him. Sacred space was created.

The elder then approaches a neighbor across the street attempting to edge her lawn with a hand tool. The elder approaches, greets the neighbor and offers to loan his power weed-wacker for this job. The neighbor, a little caught off guard, hesitates and then accepts the offer. Later when the neighbor returns the weed-wacker, the young woman and the older man find themselves planning to buy a power washer together. They come to the conclusion that each of them needn't buy equipment alone when they can split the cost. The elder suggests that they expand the agreement. If either person ends up moving out of the community, that person will receive a fair cash settlement for their ownership and leave the machine in the community. They both assume that other neighbors may want to use the power washer. The expanded relationship between the two results in the neighbor's expanded passion for sharing with other neighbors as well. Sacred space has allowed the holy practice of service. The following week, the neighbor offers to power wash the slippery sidewalk of the single mother across the cul-de-sac.

She explains to the elder that since the woman works, one of her greatest challenges is finding adequate child care. During the day she takes her children to a day care center. The remainder of the time she must often use unfamiliar babysitters so that she can get away occasionally. After confirming with his wife, the elder later visits the single mother and offers his home as a safe place for her children to stay whenever she is in a pinch. The following year, the woman and her children celebrate Thanksgiving with the elder and his wife. The children's grandparents live across the country and seldom are able to visit. Sacred space, once created, can also end up feeling like a home away from home.

Connect to others. Share with others. Serve others. This facilitates the action of community. "To commune" originally meant to be in connection with others. Once this connection exists, the people begin to set standards for living with one another that make it possible to have a higher standard of living. When people join the community, they receive the blessing of the intimately connected group. Is the Jewish boy truly confirmed if no one attends his bar mitzvah? Is a person really married if the ceremony of marriage does not include an endorsement from one's community? Entering into meaningful connection with others enriches us. Can a human being raised from birth by wolves ever develop a human personality? Can we grow into full personhood without seeing ourselves reflected in the response of others? One core of effective community is the functional family.

Advocating for Family

Families need glue to hold them together. Both extended and nuclear families are being threatened with extinction. Not more than thirty-five years ago the number of American children living apart from their biological fathers was seventeen percent of the total (Popenoe, 1996, p.191). A first marriage today has only a 50% chance of survival. Fatherlessness caused by births out-of-wedlock almost equals in number the ones caused by divorce. One kind of glue that is missing in family is father and grandfather energy. Men have an irreplaceable role to play in child development, and no social unit is more necessary in a healthy culture than the family. Grandfathers can do at least two things to strengthen the family: to maintain a commitment to the woman in their life as a model, and to be accessible to their grandchildren, especially those whose father is distant. Involved biological fathers are deeply caring and selfless toward their children. This kind of father energy can't be transferred easily. Grandfathers have more of this energy than most any other man, including stepfathers.

I am also aware of the wonderful stepfathers many of us have known. My confidence in involved genetic fatherhood is meant to emphasize the importance of genetic grandfathers. I don't want to show disdain for involved stepfathers, but rather encourage grandfathers to follow their hearts directly into the arms of their children's children. Our bias against older people has allowed them to lose confidence in their grandparent potential. The family needs this energy. Remember, to reach elder levels of maturity requires an expression of generativity, an aspect of which is an active concern for others beyond the members of one's nuclear family and for younger generations in general. The personal benefits are measurable. The happiest group of men in North America has been found to be those over age 50 living with their mate in the "empty nest" (Campbell, 1981,p.231). Could it be in part because they have access to grandchildren in a way that is both generative and delightful, and they get to see this in the eyes of the child?

The family changes as society changes, not the reverse. Urban society has intruded forcefully on the family, taking over many functions that were once the province of the family. The family is relinquishing the job of socialization of children earlier and earlier. Schools, mass media and the peer group are taking over the guidance and education of children. But society has not developed adequate sources of socialization and support to replace that which the family has relinquished. At the same time, conditions that allow or require both spouses to work outside the home create situations that can heighten and exacerbate conflict between the spouses. Action elderhood is now more necessary than ever!

I remain within reach of my adult children. It is no longer my role to be an "in your face parent," but my interdependence with my children makes it necessary for me to be accessible and available upon request. Action grandparenting in my family includes supporting both my adult children and their children. With my children's permission, I can play a role in child care, for example. A grandparent can loan money and other resources to facilitate an adult child's movement from one stage of life to another. Elder grandparents can take responsibility for maintaining family traditions like the Christmas wreath on the front door, annual trips to the pumpkin patch before Halloween and renting the cabin at the beach each August. Action grand parenting also requires allowing family traditions to be challenged and changed as your adult children grow. When my oldest son had his first children, he wanted to be at his own house, with his new family on Christmas morning. My wife and I let go of our family tradition of gathering at our home and developed with my son and his wife a new Christmas morning ritual that met his new needs and retained some of our extended family practices. He and his brood now come to our house for a late morning breakfast, thus leaving room for him to do Christmas in his way as well as ours.

Family has both internal and external functions. The internal function is the psychosocial protection and nurturing of its members. The external function is accommodation to the culture and the transmission of that culture's ideals (Minuchin, 1974, p.46). Elders usually have more credibility within their own families than they do in the wider community, so why not begin your eldering there? Action elderhood has great potential as a generative force backing up the parents of the nuclear family. The elder can, in many ways, if he or she desires, assist in the protection and nurture of the children and grandchildren. The two great social structures, extended family and culture, can act to protect and generate strong elders.

Passing It On

The elder eventually turns over family leadership to the younger members of the community. In our culture from age 55 to 75 years, we typically find professional people withdrawing from power roles such as entrepreneur and politician. In the Far East, the older man is expected to lose interest in temporal affairs and shift toward a more spiritual focus. Some primitive cultures perceive the passing of leadership to younger people as the peak of the life cycle.

The elder gradually lets go of the need for control, coordination and command. Passing on the power is an expression of the wise older person's increasing hunger for connection and simplification of their life. They want to stir the heart of community while assisting the young in their drive to make the community productive. The elder knows they are not a leader any longer. The leaders are the young whom they have raised. Margaret Mead mused, "There are no elders who know what those who have been reared within the last twenty years know about the world into which they were born" (Mead, 1970, p.61). Mead was an elder who believed that former ways of being were precursors rather than models for the leaders of the present.

The generations following the 21st Century elder will have to cope with more rapid changes in their culture than ever before. They have watched the locus of world power shift completely away from Cold War status. The means of communication and technology in general have changed enormously in their time. There were no cell phones before 1980. There were only a few computers before 1980. Even the generation Mead studied thirty-five years ago had observed the "definition of humanity, the limits of their explorable Universe, the certainties of a known and limited world, the fundamental imperatives of life and death—all change before their eyes" (Mead, 1970, p.61). To these experts in change management, the elder relinquishes control.

Modeling Good Health

The male provider, in my opinion, who is the most effective is the healthy man who lives a long life because he is as concerned with his own happiness and physical well being as he is that of those whom he loves. Ask a man whom he cares for the most, his wife or himself? It is difficult to find a man who will tell us he must first care for himself to assure he is strong enough to provide for others. This logic escapes Western men who have been taught that they are a tool of society, a "man-o-war" and a machine that moves the cogs of business and industry. They become too busy to care for themselves. Men in this culture have a tougher time keeping good care of themselves, however. Older men's health is generally worse than older women's.

American men over sixty-five commit suicide over five times more often than women in their age group. Men are more susceptible to chronic illnesses, including cancer although the rate of cancer among women has increased the past few decades. Men over sixty-five are twice as likely to become victims of violent crime as women. They are four times more likely to become hospitalized for alcohol-related problems (Kimbrell, 1995p.201). The lamentable facts about men's health show the extent to which our masculine mystique has put men in a vulnerable place. As men continue to live shorter, more stressful lives than women, the mystique infuses us with values that discourage men from doing anything to prevent poor health. "Their machine-man view of themselves and their bodies as... productive mechanisms programmed for constant performance and endless labor—..." (Kimbrell, pp.210-211) causes them to avoid good health care. Have you a "men's health clinic" in your community? It isn't likely.

Having said this, however, whether you are a male or female elder a healthy model is needed for those young people we serve. Rather than accept the bias toward aging, we can encourage those who see as examples of older people by showing them our diets are good, we are physically active and we are not obese. Elders act as providers when they influence younger men and women to take responsibility for their health. Young men and women need to see the elder getting an annual physical and visiting the dentist regularly. The elder needs to model eating a balanced diet, monitoring their cholesterol and replacing processed foods with fruits and vegetables. In this way the elder provides a model of a person who understands their mortal reality. The elderly have a fear of obsolescence and a depleted body rings the discard bell. Depletion is not seen simply as an aspect of the second half of life but rather as the end to our usefulness. The elder has a healthy and invigorating image of what an older person can be. They don't buy into the masculine or feminine mystique or the biases about aging in America. They provide hope for younger people about both maturity and the credibility of a balanced older person.

Protector Roles for Elders

The mature expression of protector is not as much a hero as a balance of warrior, magician, sovereign and lover. Although heroes are courageous, in Western tradition they have been emotionally mute and invulnerable. They lack transparency and are solitary people. We can understand this even better by remembering that both men and women are protectors. Mature elders of both genders balance aspects of the four archetypes in their expression of the role of protector. From warrior energy they develop a commitment to a cause larger than themselves that serves others. From magician energy they gain healer power utilizing insight and reflection to assess the needs of others. From lover energy they find passion and connection through feeling. From sovereign energy they have a hunger to affirm others and to restore order from social chaos.

Up through the 20th Century, we raised our sons to believe that a protector must take hazardous risks and accept challenges that could cause them physical and emotional injury. Being courageous often meant denying fear and plunging into high-risk situations. The 21st Century elder protects by calling on our feminine energy more and becoming models of stewardship for people and Earth. They model advocacy for people without hope and perpetuate nondiscrimination. We will find the elders who have a balance of feminine and masculine expression involved in social action including both volunteer work and political activity. They model nonviolence in their careful use of media, especially television. They protect by leaving a legacy of hope for younger generations. Their legacy is a demonstration that the second half of life is for growth, transformation, healing and service. They beseech their Supreme Being to use them as a vessel for the blessing of the children.

Stewardship

Magician energy fosters harmony with nature. When we balance this with the ordering inclination of the sovereign, the assertiveness of the warrior and the awareness of the oneness of all things that comes from the lover, we have stewardship. The steward is the keeper, entrusted with the affairs of others for whom he is the advocate. You will recall in Chapter II how indigenous cultures almost universally assume that human beings are responsible for sustaining harmony in nature. The elders who were most respected by primitive people were those who understood the orderly and harmonious whole of the Universe. Older people are usually more interested in conservation than are the young. They remember the woods near their home in which they could play in a way that is more filled with awe.

How does the elder turn his concern for Earth into stewardship? Let's take a walk once again through the community and watch what the action elder does. We find the elder near their home returning from a walk with a flattened beer can in hand. The elder found it on the road, and knew it did not contribute to the beauty of our surroundings. The elder recycled it. Next, we find the elder calling the local curbside recycling company. The elder discovers that they will accept not only newspapers, but also the tons of junk mail he/she used to throw into the garbage can. The elder tells the neighbors about the news, and they spread the word.

Once again, action elderhood does not require a time consuming volunteer commitment. There are small behaviors that provide a service while at the same time model advocacy for people and Earth. Action elderhood is living the role of steward as naturally and spontaneously as possible. There are certainly much larger steps a steward of Earth can take, such as replanting and supporting conservationist organizations. My focus here is to affirm life in the simplest ways at first and then watch and see where it takes me. When elders behave this way, they model hope that the ecological destruction we have witnessed in our lifetime can be balanced at least a little, right within our community. When the action elder creates hope by this action their behavior is sacred. Religious, political and scientific leaders from eighty-three nations met a few years ago and declared:

> As scientists many of us have had profound experiences of awe and reverence before the universe. We understood that what is regarded as sacred is more likely to be treated with care and respect. Our planetary home should be so regarded. Efforts to safeguard and cherish the environment need to be infused with a vision of the sacred. (Suzuki, 1992, p.227)

In their day-to-day life, elders show care for their family and community as well as the larger community of living organisms with whom they share Earth.

A Soul Nourishing Pace

Another way the elder protects is by demonstrating ways in which the lifegiving breath, or soul, can be nourished. This is a purpose of their spiritual journey. Our soul is actualized in human ways that reflect a person's awe of creation, the love of others, gratitude and the celebration I call harvesting. There are simple yet effective ways that an elder can model soul nourishment.

In this fast moving culture, we have taken for granted a number of behaviors that starve the soul. One of the most common is watching television and going to movie theaters indiscriminately. At the elder's house, the young will find evidence of discernment in what they will watch on TV. Our willingness to indulge in violence and exploitation in entertainment media is one price we pay for haste. The elder has slowed their pace and searches the television for messages of joy, reflection and commitment that are worth viewing. The elder's grandchildren aren't allowed to play violent video games in the elder's home. The children find a warmth and fun loving spirit in the elder's home that makes up for the restrictions. They are able to consider an alternative approach to the use of media.

As the elder walks their contemplative pace in the community, they extend the boundary of sacred space. My youngest son worked in a fast food restaurant at the counter, serving customers. At age sixteen he was already aware that rude and aggressive customers acted the way they did because of the pressure of time. Fast food is a ubiquitous option in culinary pursuit in our culture despite its unhealthy nature. We rush in, hardly notice the young human beings working for low wages, grumble an order, complain in a way that does not show common sense, then rush to eat in our automobiles with one hand and take cellular phone calls with the other. My son said it was an uncommon delight when a customer with a patient smile made it clear that their priority was the connection they made with him. The elder models a response to customer service that I call *customer receptivity*. The core of customer receptivity is the recognition by the customer that the person serving him or her also wants to be seen and acknowledged. The elder models customer receptivity as he or she waits patiently to be served focused first on the person serving and second on the service they are buying. The elder knows that errors made in the customer service process are human errors made on the human journey that are to be expected with patience and generosity.

The elder nourishes us by truly seeing us as we go about performing our work. Elders accomplish these things by discovering the pace of life that fits them. They show us how we can nourish our own soul if only we take the time to smell the roses. In the 1930's, when Hans Selye outlined the first major theory of stress management, he taught that humans have a limited amount of adaptability energy. He asserted that we have a pool of energy unique to each of us. The effective stress manager learns their capacity and develops practices that allow them to live within that pool. If we don't honor our pool of energy and overuse it, we age too quickly because some of the energy we burn up is not replenishable.

Measuring our pace is a practice that allows us to remain within our pool of adaptability energy. Watch elders. They harvest their lives in part by living within their pool of energy, by understanding the limits of their knowledge and by not exposing themselves to stressors that over-tax their emotional energy. Then, "A natural enfoldment takes place...which signals a certain time when the accumulated wisdom of a lifetime reaches the state of overflow. Awakened to elderhood, we pour the distillate of our lives into other vessels, an act that not only seeds the future, but that crowns our lives with worth and nobility" (Schachter-Shalomi, 1995, p.190). Elders do this not only for their own sake, but also because of their generative concern for the welfare of those who might consider them mentors, and as a model to younger generations.

Protecting Through Blessing

The unfolding of wisdom, the pouring of the distillate of our lives into younger vessels is both a form of blessing and a transmission. By the time my second grandchild was born, I felt a need rise in me to bless her on behalf of the older people in the family. I felt the opportunity and the obligation of grand fatherhood. It was vague, but I believe I was standing in as the representative of my ancestors. I had an opportunity to pass the family name on to my granddaughter, tell her the stories of our generation and share stories about the time before my lifetime. In these ways I transmit a blessing. To accomplish all of this, I needed to bring focus to my granddaughter by creating a ritual of initiation that endorsed her as the newest member of the family.

You will recall how, when we reviewed the belief system of older cultures in Chapter II, many believed that in the second half of life we begin to connect metaphysically with our ancestors. This is one reason why older people are shown such deference in China, for example. Older

Chinese men who have pulled back from leadership of society are inclined to move forward to the "spiritual perimeter [of the culture], to confront the powerful and empowering gods. Older men discover in the supernaturals the strength that they no longer find within themselves... they use prayer...to beseech for themselves and for the people, their fire from the gods" (Gutmann, 1994, p.221). These "gods" include ancestors who now dwell with God. When my granddaughter came into the world, she was very close to God and "the gods" having recently come from within their midst. As I connected to her in the ceremony my wife and I created, I was completing a circle: we come from the Universe into this life carrying with us the knowledge of our godliness; then we grow, forgetting our source and seek the meaning of our existence; then in the second half of life we begin approaching death, the end of life, and become a connection to all who came before and will ever be.

Now I seek out opportunities to be a transmitter and source of blessing in the family. Holiday meals are good opportunities to utilize elder energies of blessing. The blessing ceremonies my wife and I sponsored for my children are now models my children may emulate. I plan to attend the baptisms, bat mitzvahs and any religious ceremonies honoring my grandchildren to boost the ritual with grandfather energy. My granddaughter's ceremony was simple to create. My wife and I went to my granddaughter's home, and with her parents' permission we did three things. First, we spoke to my granddaughter, who was one week old, about our appreciation for her existence in our life. I affirmed in front of my son and daughter-in-law my vision of the baby's future using words like healthy, successful and happy. Next, I anointed her forehead with a consecrated olive oil a friend had brought to me from Israel. As I touched the baby, I made a verbal commitment to her that I would help her realize her future and her dream. And finally, my wife and I gave her a small cross on a chain that her parents will keep for her to wear when she is old enough.

I really didn't know anything about formal blessings as I put together the ceremony, and I felt clumsy doing it. The endorsement I got from my son's eyes, however, made it all seem right. How can a grandfather fail in blessing if he is in love with his grandchild? From Chapter I you will recall that a blessing has five parts: Touch; Special words; An expression of appreciation for one being blessed; A reference to supporting the blessed one's dream for the future; and An active commitment to the one being blessed to help them realize their dream.

The blessing is a divination that the one being blessed need not either accept or understand. It is the elder's declaration before his or her community, in sacred space, of commitment to the one being blessed. My granddaughter may never be told that she received this blessing. I believe, nevertheless, that the affirmation in the blessing experience moves the energy of the Universe to bring support and vigor to her.

The aged were powerful in many ancient societies. Their special stature had to do with their privileged access to the supernatural. Whether we believe in the idea of blessing or not, elders carry a responsibility to both transmit information to the young and to stand ready to serve them as they venture on their journey. If not through blessing, elders will hopefully find some way to assure the young that they are available to them and they passionately care about their success.

Heeding Those Without Hope

As I mentioned above, the creation of sacred space begins when one person is seen by another. The homeless, unemployed, disabled and other victims of our prejudice can begin a move away and out of economic and mental poverty if more of us were willing to see them. The elder, moving with *thanatos* energy, sees the homeless. Elders see them much like they see themselves. They were born just like everyone else, to a mother in a place called home and had a father or longed for one. Like themselves the elders see the homeless are embodied spirits, sparks of God. That ties us together with them. Like the elder, they need to be seen. Many hopeless men, women and children would add that the ruin of homes begins in the heart of the father. Remembering the statistics about fatherlessness and that nearly one-third of children are born out of wedlock in the USA, the elder shivers at what the statistic must be for the poor, the homeless and minorities.

Black activist and scholar W.E.B. DuBois wrote in 1912, "Ought children be born to us? Have we a right to make human souls face what we face today? The answer is clear: if the great battle of human right against poverty, against color prejudice is to be won, it must be won not in our day, but in the day of our children's children" (DuBois, 1964, p.44). The elders know they must depend on the next generation to do the next great work in society. Like DuBois, the elders expect to be supportive to the social activists among the young and know their responsibility is to hold the container for them, rather than lead the great battle of human rights themselves. How does the elder hold the container for the advocates of the hopeless? Let's take it in levels of intensity of involvement.

Increasing Levels of Elder Action

Let's say there are four levels of intensity to the role of an action elder. At the first level of action elderhood elders *see* the homeless or the victim of discrimination. They know they are seen because in first level action the hopeless hear the elder say, "May I help you?" or "Do you know of a place you can sleep tonight?" because the elders know how to find shelters in their city. Driving in a suburban area recently I saw a man walking in the rain with no shoes or hat. I was in a hurry and continued on so that I would be on time for something I thought was more important. I didn't even express first level action because I didn't take the opportunity to really see the man.

In level two actions if I was calling on my elder within I might have done this instead: Once I saw the man I would have stopped my car at the next public phone and call whoever was expecting met to report that I would be a little late for the appointment. I would then have taken my umbrella, left my car, crossed the street and walked to where the shoeless man was standing saying, "Pardon me; I see that you have no shoes. Would you allow me to help you find a pair?" From this point forward, it would be the shoeless man's right to respond any way that he wished. If he accepts the offer, the two of us could arrange to meet somewhere safe for both after I found some shoes that will fit the man. The elder needn't take big risks like giving the needy a ride in their car or inviting them into their home. The act of approaching the man connects the two at the heart and builds sacred space.

Level three actions on behalf of the hopeless would include offering your time to the organizations that seek to improve the lives of unemployed, minority, disabled, imprisoned and homeless people. You will find that the United Way, churches and charitable organizations need mature, impassioned people as advisors and sources of leadership. Most of these groups are governed by boards of volunteer directors made up of people who are folks like you and I. We need nothing but time and interest to qualify. Because of the management and advocacy of these directors, organizations are funded that employ DuBois's children's children, who do the level four work in the trenches. DuBois went on to say that the reason our children are on the frontline is that the elders have on them the "blood and dust of battle," and for the young, "theirs the rewards of victory" won in our early efforts to free the hopeless. "If they are not there [doing our level four work], because we have not brought them to the world, then we have been the guiltiest factor in conquering ourselves" (Dubois, p.44).

Don't let me discourage you from level four action by suggesting that it is primarily the work of the next generation. I want to inspire you to consider yourself a natural resource. It is possible, however, to be a natural resource and to take action in small ways. North Americans, more than most peoples believe in the potential of what one person can do. If we start with a smile, an extended moment of accessibility, or a gift of a pair of shoes, then anyone can play a part in action elderhood. Consider September 11, 2001, however. What was the role of elders that day? The heroes of the day were the young and we would have expected that. Elders can do a lot of level one, two and three work, however.

Throughout time older people have demonstrated a desire to have an impact. Retirement and disengagement from the community was not the manner of elders in early world history. In a survey done of older people in over seventy pre-industrial societies worldwide, gerontologist Leo Simmons found five recurring, primary interests. One, to live a long life, second, to increase time available for relaxation, third, to hold on to rights that come with seniority, fourth, to withdraw from life at its end with honor, fifth, "To remain participants in the affairs of life in either operational or supervisory roles, any sharing in group interests being preferred to idleness and indifference" (Simmons, 1945, P.50). The urge to be visible, accessible and potent and to serve is hard-wired into all of us.

We all admire elders who have excelled at level four action. Nelson Mandella, Betty Ford, Georgia O'Keefe, Benjamin Spock and others have modeled level four action at an older age than most activists. If we are ready, we can sit with dying AIDS patients in a hospice, build dikes against flooding rivers, counsel boys in gangs on the street, mentor drug abusers in a drop-in center, tutor children with reading problems, deliver food to the poor and do hands-on political campaigning. The balanced elder integrates the reflective energy of *thanatos* with the creative energy of *libido*. *Libido* still drives us in the second half of life. For some people this energy remains at a high level throughout life. The wonderful reality about the sage is that we can all depend on them to make good judgments about how they use their energy.

Elders As Teachers

Men and women share the third traditional parent role of teacher of cultural tradition. Up until the Industrial Revolution, parents taught the young how to survive and, as an extension of that, how to protect their family. This included teaching crafts, skills with tools and skills with weapons. In the 18th Century, with the advent of public school systems, parents were teachers of knowledge, of comportment and of the governing of the community. In the 19th Century men modeled how to work for a wage in addition to working to create products of living and trade. They taught how to build and maintain corporations. In the 20th Century both men and women coach and guide others to be successful in the professions and in the trades.

Elders of the 21st Century seed the future in their teaching role. They are mentors, storytellers and wisdomkeepers who stand ready to serve the young people who seek them out. They model "following your own bliss" while at the same time seeking out young people to improve the success of their journey.

Passing On A Legacy

Rabbi Schacter-Shalomi says that to leave a legacy is to be *saved* to the hard drive of your community's memory. If we buy into the American aging model of retirement, our long life experience can be lost to the generations that follow. Successful aging, then, means more vital involvement for the elder who is sageing, while at the same time being a resource to others. The sage, the elder as mentor, wants to leave a legacy because they have confidence in what life has taught them. If a person follows the traditional retirement model of late life expression, it might suggest that they lack confidence in their wisdom because retirement is not about leaving a legacy. Retirement has become our word for getting away and getting out of the way and avoiding passing it on before we pass on.

Reaching Out to Younger People

To come of age, to come to maturity, a young male or female needs models. They need models of both feminine and masculine expression in both older men and older women. They need to see the four archetypes balanced in their mentors' expression. "When we stand physically close to our father, something—something moves over that can't be described in material terms..." (Bly, 1990). And it goes both ways, for a person can't possibly know what all of life means until they have a child or experience the love of a child. In fact it is our children's expectations of parents that make a father and mother become their best. The most mature role a person will play is parent. All of us can have an impact on children, however, whether we parent them or not.

Take a few minutes and make a list of the people, who, to any extent, had a positive influence on you. My piano teacher was in my life twice a month. Her sensitive manner and her respect for me caused me to love the piano. My best friend in my senior class in high school once told me he didn't feel I showed adequate respect for a girl I dated. He was my first morality coach. The man who was my first management-consulting customer was the labor relations coordinator for a paper mill. He modeled for me a passion for a quality work life. He was extraordinarily patient with the managers of the mill that he needed to confront in ongoing negotiations. Doug, the elder I told you about in Chapter I, was obese. He did not model perfection, but he walked in the world with a love for others that was incomparable. It was a kind of summons to the heart of the other.

Some of us are blessed with numerous mentors. All of us were touched by a few. I met an eighty-year-old man who told me he could not recall ever having a mentor. He was an unhappy man and his unhappiness was compounded by his inability to recognize anyone who held his dream. He also had chosen to miss out on the experience of being a mentor to others, as well. Mentoring is the giving of a blessing to the person for whom we are the advocate. Blessings are given in subtle ways including touch, the use of special words and a look that really sees the one being blessed. "Looking back, I realize that I was blessed with mentors at every crucial stage of my young life, but a funny thing happened on the way to full adulthood: the mentors stopped coming. For several years I waited for the next one in vain..." (Palmer, 1998, p.25). This writer realized in the second half of life that it was now time for him to become a mentor.

A few places where older and younger people meet are worth mentioning. The scouting programs in North America not only connect men and boys, women and girls, but also offer rites of passage. The increasingly demanding challenge of moving higher and higher in the ranks of scouting is an initiation into adulthood. The Service Corps of Retired Executives, SCORE, provides free advice to young business people. Over 13,000 retired business managers, entrepreneurs and professionals donate almost unlimited time to the task of advising on the manner in which we form a new business. The Small Business Administration of the US government sponsors the program. The Big Brothers and The Big Sisters, two of America's oldest and largest mentoring programs, can't find enough qualified people who will volunteer. Studies have shown that boys with mentors in Big Brothers are forty-six percent less likely to begin using drugs and fifty-two percent are less likely to skip school. All of these programs need more participation from mature men and women.

The biggest demand for action elderhood, however, is inside your personal sphere of influence — family, community, church and workplace. It is likely that most of the people inside your sphere will not expect action elderhood from you. That is why I suggest that the aspiring elder move into action in small ways at first, developing the roles of provider, protector and teacher gradually. The process might begin with increasing your accessibility and then moving to some minor community advocacy such as donating blood to the Red Cross or beginning a dialogue with the neighbors we have not gotten to know. No matter how elder like we presently are in our extended family, this is where we are probably going to find the most opportunity for action elderhood. How much preparation have we made to offer leadership to the young members of our family? Are we trying our best to take care of ourselves so that we model the fourfold balance of physical, mental, intellectual and spiritual being? Have we begun to supervise the collection of family historical artifacts? Are we a source of blessing at family gatherings?

As we grow in confidence, we will seek ways to develop our elder role. This requires not only a demonstrated concern for people, community and Earth, but increased movement in the direction of those who need our advocacy and our blessing. Gradually, the family will begin to notice our soul nourishing pace and lifestyle. "Where is grandma?" one child will say to another. "Oh, I think she is meditating again," reports the other grandchild, with both pride and a little embarrassment. We will find that we have an increasing tendency to look out for others, see them and desire to give a little of our time. It doesn't matter whether we behave with level one, two, three or four actions. What matters is that we look increasingly for ways to affirm life. It is this hunger that brings out the wisdomkeeper in an elder.

The move away from the doingness of our earlier years into the beingness of the second half of life does not mean that elders are passive. Being is a calling to the being in others, a resonance with others. Elder being is a state of accessibility and a passion for celebration of long life, service, and an inner intimacy with your eternal spirit. Elder being is an understanding of mortality, the spiritual journey and an earnest concern for the quality of life on this planet. Elder being is a restoration of ancient human's uncontrollable commitment to cultivating and sowing the next generation—*from the heart.*

References

A Gathering of Men (1990), Video interview by Bill Moyers of Robert Bly.

Adams, Frances (1972). The Role of Old People in Santo Tomas Mazaltepec. PP.103-26. In Cowgill, Donald O. and Holmes, L.D. Editors. *Aging and Modernization*. New York. Appleton-Century-Crofts.

Albom, Mitch(1997). *Tuesdays With Morrie*. New York. Doubleday.

Alcohol Problems Prevalent Among Elderly. Washington Post, Sept. 8, 1993. P.A5 quoted in Andrew Kimbrell (1995). *The Masculine Mystique*. New York. Ballantine Books.

Allred, Wayne(1996). *Geezerhood*. Roy, Utah.Willow Tree Books.

Archenbaum, W. Andrews (1986). The Aging of the First New Nation. In Alan Pfizer and Lydia Bronte, Eds. *Our Aging Society*. New York.WW Norton Co.

Aristotle (1959). *The Ethics*. Trans. J.A.K. Thomson. New York. Harmondsworth. IV.I; VIII. 3-6.

Arrien, Angeles (1998). *The Second Half of Life*. Boulder, Colo. Sounds True tape series.

Augustine (1945). Enarrationes in Psalmos. 112.2 In Erich Przywara, Editor. *An Augustine Synthesis*. New York. Steed and Ward.

Berry, Thomas and Brian Swimme (1992). *The UniverseStory*. HarperSanFrancisco.

Bianchi, Eugene (1982). *Aging as a Spiritual Journey*. New York. Crossroad.

Bly, Robert (1990). *Iron John*. New York.Vintage Books.

Bolen, Jean Shinoda(2003). *Crones Don't Whine*. Boston. Conari Press.

Bolen, Jean Shinoda (2001). *Goddesses in Older Women*. New York. HarperCollins Pub.

Borg, Marcus J (1994). *Meeting Jesus Again for the First Time*. HarperSanFrancisco.

Hildegard of Bingen (1997). Quoted in *The Oxford Dictionary of World Religions*.Editor, John Bowker. Oxford U. Press.

Buber, Martin (1967). The Disciple. In *A Believing Humanism*. New York.Simon and Schuster.

Buber, Martin (1958). *To Hallow This Life*. New York. Harper and Brothers Pub.

Bunzel, Ruth(1932). Introduction to Zuni Ceremonialism. Wash. D.C. *44th Annual Report of the Bureau of American Ethnology*. P. 516-17.

Butler, Robert M., M.D (1974). Successful Aging and the Role of Life Review. In Journal of the American Geriatrics Society. Vol. XXII. No. 12. P. 534.

Campbell, Angus (1981). *The Sense of Well Being in America*. New York. McGraw-Hill.

Campbell, Joseph (1970). *Myths to Live By*. New York. Bantam Books.

Chapman, Elwood (1986). *Comfort Zones: Planning Your Future*. New York. W.W.Norton and Co.

Chinen, Allan (1989). *In The Ever After*. Wilmette, Illinois. Chiron Pub.

Cohen, Gene D. MD (2000). *The Creative Age*. New York. HarperCollins Pub.

Conroy, Pat (1995). *Beach Music*. New York. Doubleday.

Cook, Shelburne (1972). Aging of and in Populations. P.S. Timiras, Editor. New York *Developmental Physiology and Aging*.

Copleston, F (1947). *A History of Philosophy*. New York. Vol, 8. Part II. P. 20.

Cowgill, Donald O (1986). *Aging Around the World*. Belmont, California. Wadsworth Pub. Co.

Curran, Charles E (1985). Aging: A Theological Perspective. In Carol LeFevre and LeFevre, *Aging and the Human Spirit*. New York. Exploration Pr.

de Beauvoir, Simone (1972). *The Coming of Age*. New York. GP Putnam's Sons.

References

de Beauvoir, Simone (1977). *Old Age.* New York. Harmondsworth.

Demos, John (1986). *Past, Present and Personal: The Family and Life Course in American History.* Oxford U. Press.

Dewey, J. and J.H. Tufts (1913). *Ethics.* New York. Harcourt Press.

Donne, John (1952). Death's Duell or, a Consolation to the Soule, Against the Dying Life, and Living Death of the Body. In *The Complete Poetry and Selected Prose of John Doone.* Editor: Charles M. Coffin. New York. Random House.

Dublin, Thomas (1979). *Women at Work.* New York. Columbia U. Press.

Du Bois, W.E.B (1964). *An ABC of Color.* New York. International Pub.

Dychtwald, Ken (1990). *Age Wave.* New York. Bantam Books.

(1997) *Meister Eckhart: The Essential Writings.* Quoted in The Oxford Dictionary of World Religions. Ed. Bowker, John. Oxford U. Press.

Eisler, Riane (1995). *The Chalice and the Blade.* HarperSanFrancisco.

Eliade, Mircea (1958). *Rites and symbols of initiation.* New York. Harper and Row.

Eliade, Mircea (1959). *The Sacred and the Profane: The Nature of Religion: The Significance Of Religious Myth, Symbolism and Ritual Within Life and Culture.* New York. Harcourt Brace Jovanovich.

Encyclopedia Britannica Deluxe Edition, 2004 Cd-ROM.

Erasmus (1974). *Praise of Folley.*Translated by Betty Radice. London.

Erikson, Eric (1986). *Vital Involvement In Old Age.* New York. W.W. Norton & Co.

Erikson, Erik H (1950). *Childhood and Society.* New York. W.W. Norton and Co.

Estes, Clarissa, Ph.D (19920. *Women Who Run With Wolves.* New York. Ballantine Books.

Farrell, Warren (1993). *The Myth of Male Power.* New York. Simon and Schuster.

Fenner, Elizabeth (1995). Sizing Up The Risks of Living Together. In *Money*. July, 1995.

Fischer, David H (1978). *Growing Old in America*. New York. Oxford U. Press.

Fischer, Kathleen (1995). *Autumn Gospel*. New York. Integration Books.

Foster, Steven and Meredith Little (1992). *The Book of the Vision Quest*. New York. Fireside.

Foster, Steven and Meredith Little (1984). *The Trail to the Sacred Mountain*. Big Pine, California. Lost Borders Press.

Fox, Matthew (1983b). *The Coming of the Cosmic Christ*. Harper and Row. San Francisco.

Fox, Matthew (1991). *Creation Spirituality*. HarperSanFrancisco.

Fox, Matthew (2002). *Creativity*. New York. Jeremy P. Tarcher.

Fox, Matthew (1983a). *Original Blessing*. New York. Jeremy P. Tarcher/ Putnam.

Fox, Matthew (1995). *The Reinvention of Work*. HarperSanFrancisco.

Fox, Matthew (1990). *Spirituality Named Compassion*. Rochester, Vermont. Inner Traditions.

Fox, Robin (1975). *Encounter With Anthopology*. London. Peregrine.

France, Peter (1996). *Hermits*. New York. St. Martin's Press.

Furstenberg, Frank and Christine W. Nord (1985). Parenting Apart: Patterns of Childbearing After Marital Disruption. In Journal of Marriage and the Family. 47(4): PP. 893-905.

Gandhi, Mahatma (1984). *All Men Are Brothers*. New York. The Continuum Publishing Corporation.

Gennep, Arnold Van (1960). *The Rites of Passage*. U. of Chicago Press. Translation of Gennep's 1908, Les rites de passage.

Gibran Kahlil (1951). *The Prophet*. New York. Alfred A. Knopf.

Goldberg, Herb (1976). *The Hazards of Being Male*. New York. New American Library.

(1926). Grant Kalendrier et compost des bergiers. 1500 edition. Quoted by J. Morawski. *Les douze mois figurez.* In Archivum Romanicum. P. 351.

Gurdjieff, G.I (1969). *Meetings With Remarkable Men.* New York: E.P. Dutton.

Gutmann, David (1994). *Reclaimed Powers.* Evanston, Illinois. Northwestern U. Press. Evanston, III.

Hammond, J.L. and Barbara (1912). *The Village Laborer, 1760-1832.* London: Longmans Green. Quoted in Kimbrell.

Harkness, Helen (1999). Don't Stop the Career Clock. Palo Alto, California. Davies-Black Publishing.

Harvey, Andrew (1994). *The Way of Passion.* Berkeley, California. Frog,Ltd.

Heard, Gerald (1963). *The Five Ages of Man.* New York. The Julian Press.

Helliwell, Tanis (1999). *Take Your Soul To Work.* Random House of Canada.

Hesse, Hermann (1951). *Siddartha.* New York. New Directions.

Hillman, James (1987). Senex and Puer. In *Puer Papers.* Editor. James Hillman. Dallas. Spring Publications.

Hillman, James (1999)). *The Force of Character.* New York. Ballantine Books.

Hildegard of Bingen (1997). Quoted in *The Oxford Dictionary of World Religions.*Editor, John Bowker. Oxford U. Press.

Iser, Lynne, compiler (1996). *The Spiritual Eldering Workbook.* Boulder, Colorado. Spiritual Eldering Institute.

Johnson, Elizabeth (1992). *She Who Is* .New York. Crossroad.

Jones, Terry (2005). *Elder as Revived Child.* Unpublished poem.

Jones, Terry (2001). *The Elder Within.* Wilsonville, Oregon. Bookpartners.

Joseph, Jenny (1991). *When I Am An Old Woman I Shall Wear Purple.* Watsonville, California. Papier-Mache Press.

Jung, Carl (1971). Joseph Campbell, Editor. *The Portable Jung.* New York. Penguin Books.

Kauth, Bill (1992). *A Circle of Men.* New York. St. Martin's Press.

Khan, H.I (1964). *The Sufi Message of Hazrat Inayat Khan.* Vol. X. London. Barrie and Jenkins.

Kimbrell, Andrew (1995). *The Masculine Mystique.* New York. Ballantine Books.

Kimura, Doreen (1992). Sex Difference in the Brain In *Scientific American.* September. 119-125.

Klaus, Marshall and Kennell, John (1976). *Maternal-infant Bonding.* St. Louis.

Kotre, John and Elizabeth Hall (1990). *Seasons of Life.* Boston. Little, Brown and Co.

Kurtz,Gary (Producer) (1997). *StarWars.* 20th Century Fox. California.

Laffin, John (1986). *Brassey's Battles: 3500 Years of Conflict, Campaigns and Wars From A to Z.* London: A Wheaton and Co.

LaGravenese, Richard. (Producer) (1991). *The Fisher King.* California. TriStar, Hill/Obst Productions.

Lake, Robert (1990). An Indian Father's Plea. *Teacher Magazine.* Vol. 2. No. 1.P. 50.

Larue, Gerald A (1992). *Gero-Ethics.* New York. Prometheus Books.

Leder, Drew (1997). *Spiritual Passages.* New York. Jeremy P. Tarcher/Putnam.

Leslie, Gerald R. and Sheila K. Korman (1989). *The Family in Social Context.* Oxford U. Press.

Levant, Ronald F (1996). The New Psychology of Men. *Professional Psychology Research and Practice.* Vol. 27. No.3.

Levinson, Daniel J (1978). *The Seasons of a Man's Life.* New York. Ballantine Books.

Lowen, Alexander MD (1975). *Bioenergetics.* New York. Coward, McCann and Geoghegan, Inc.

Lowry, Hunt (Producer) (1995). *First Knight.* Zucker Bros. Productions. California. Columbia.

Mahdi, Louise, Foster, Stephen and Meredith Little (1987). *Betwixt and Between: Patterns of Masculine and Feminine Initiation.* LaSalle, Illinois. Open Court.

Malinowski, Bronislaw (1962). *Sex, Culture and Myth.* New York. Harcourt, Brace and World.

Marcel, Gabriel (1955). *The Decline of Wisdom.* New York. Philosophical Library.

Mathews, Mitford M (1951) *Dictionary of Americanism on Historical Principles.* U. of Chicago Press. Vol. 2. P. 1793.

Mead, Margaret (1970). *Culture and Commitment.* New York. Natural History Press/Doubleday and Co., Inc.

Mead, Margaret (1949). *Male and Female.* New York. William Morrow and Co.

Miller, Alice (1990). *The Untouched Key: Tracing Childhood Trauma in Creativity and Destructiveness.* New York. Doubleday.

Miller, Patricia H (1989). *Theories of Developmental Psychology.* .New York. W.H. Freeman and Co.

Miller, Sven (2001). *Peter Pan:Puer at Senex.* Irondale Ensemble Project News. Fall, 2001. Retrieved August 20, 2003. www.irondale.org/newsletters/Peter%20Pan/senex.htm.

Minuchin, Salvador (1974). *Families and Family Therapy.* Cambridge, Mass. Harvard U. Press.

Modell, John, Fran F. Furstenberg Jr. and Strong, Douglas (1978). The Timing of Marriage In The Transition to Adulthood: Continuity and Change, 1860-1975. In *American Journal of Sociology.* Vol. IV.

Moir, Anne and Jessel, David(1992). Brain Sex. In *Behavioral Endocrinology.* Cambridge, MA: MIT Press/Bradford Books.

Moore, Robert and Gillette, Douglas (1990). *King, Warrior, Magician, Lover: Rediscovering the Archetypes of the Mature Masculine.* San Francisco. Harper.

Moore, Robert and Douglas Gillette (1993a). *The Lover Within.* New York. William Morrow and Co.

Moore, Robert and Douglas Gillette (1993b). *The Magician Within.* San Francisco. Harper.

Morrison, Dorothy (1999). *In Praise of the Crone.* . St. Paul, Minnesota. Llewellyn Publications.

Myss, Caroline (1996). *Anatomy of the Spirit.* New York. Harmony Books.

Nachmanovitch, Stephen (1990). *Free Play.* Jeremy P. Tarcher/Putnam.

Palmer, Parker(1998). *The Courage to Teach.* San Francisco. Jossey-Bass Inc. Pub.

Parke, Ross D (1981). *Fathers.* Cambridge. Harvard U. Press.

Piaget, Jean (1967). *The Child's Conception of the World.* Totowa, New Jersey. Littlefield, Adams and Co.

Pintauro, Joseph and Sister Corita (1968). *To Believe in God.* New York. Harper and Row Pub.

Plutarch (1989). Whether an old man should engage in public affairs? *Moralia.* X. "Old men in public affairs." 784. P. 81. Quoted in Minois. *History of Old Age.*

Polanyi, Karl(1957). *The Great Transformation.* Boston. Beacon Press.

Popenoe, David (1996). *Life Without Fathers.* New York. The Free Press.

Preece, Rob (1996). *Individuation or Institution.* Mudra Publications. November 26. Retrieved November 27, 2003 from www.mudra.co.uk/mudraindividuation.html.

www.redhatsociety.com

(1992). Preserving and Cherishing the Earth: An Appeal For Joint Commitment in Science and Religion. Moscow. 1991. Quoted in David Suzuki and Peter Knudtson. *Wisdom of the Elders.* Bantam Books. New York.

Reif, Jennifer and Haleff, Marline (2003). *The Magical Crone.* New York. Citadel Press.

Reiner, Rob (Producer) (1995). *The American President*. Castle Rock, California. Wildwood Enterprises Inc, Universal.

Rich, Adrienne (1976). *Of Woman Born*. New York. W.W. Norton and Co.

Rinpoche, Sogyal (1993). *The Tibetan Book of the Living and Dying*. San Francisco. Harper.

Rotundo, E. Anthony (1985). American Fatherhood: A Historical Perspective. In *American Behavioral Scientist*. Vol. 29. No. 1. (Sept./Oct.): P. 7-25.

St. Jerome (1987). Letters. Letter XIV. Quoted in George Minois. *History of Old Age*. U. of Chicago Press.

Schachter-Shalomi, Rabbi Zalman (1995). *Age-ing to Sage-ing*. New York. Warner Books.

Schor, Juliet B (1992). *The Overworked American*. New York. Harper Collins.

Shakespeare, William (1928). As You Like It. In *The Annotated Shakespeare*. Vol. I. The Comedies. Editor, A.L. Rouse. New York. Longmeadow Press.

Silverstein, Olga and Rashbaum, Beth (1994). *The Courage to Raise Good Men*. New York. Penguin Books.

Simmons, Leo (1945). *The Role of the Aged in Primitive Society*. London. Oxford U. Press.

Smalley Gary and Trent, John (1990). *Blessing*. Tape cassette. Pocket Books.

Spyri, Joanna (1984). *Heidi*. New York. Ariel Books/Alfred A. Knopf. Ibid.

Suzuki, David and Knudtson, Peter (1992). *Wisdom of the Elders*. New York. Bantam Books.

Taylor, A.E. *Socrates* (1953). Garden City, New York. Doubleday.

Thompson, E.P (1963). *The Making of the English Working Class*. New York. Vintage Books.

Thoreau, Henry David (1980). *Walden*. New York. Signet Classics Edition.

Thurman, Howard (1965). *The Luminous Darkenss*. Richmond, Indiana. Friends United Press.

Thurman, Howard (1971). *The Search for Common Ground*. Richmond, Indiana. Friends United Press.

Tolle, Eckhart (1999). *Practicing the Power of Now*. Novato, California. New World Library.

Tolkein, J.R.R (1965a). *Fellowship of the Ring*. New York. Ballantine.

Tolkein, J.R.R (1965b). *Return of the King*. New York. Ballantine.

Tolkein, J.R.R (1965c). *The Two Towers*. New York. Ballantine.

Turner, Frederick G (1962). Middle Western Pioneer Democracy(1918). In *The Frontier in American History*. New York. Rinehart and Winston.

(1993) Dept. of Health and Human Services. Sept. 9, Vol. 9,30. Advance Report of the Final Mortality Statistics, 1991. Vol. 42. No.3. Hyattsville, Maryland. *Supplement, Monthly Vital Statistics Report*.

Vaillant, George E. MD (2002). *Aging Well*. New York. Little, Brown and Co.

Valentinus, Basilius (2004). In www.greenspirit.org/uk/resources.Four Paths.html.

Van Gennep, Arnold (1960). *The Rites of Passage*. U. of Chicago Press.

Wells, H.G (1920). *The Outline of History*. Vol. II. New York. Garden City Books.

Whitmont. E.C (1969). *The Symbolic Quest*. London. Barrie and Rockliff.

Xenophon (1910). Memorabilia of Socrates. In *Socratic Discourse Plato and Xenophon*. London. Everyman's Library.

Zukav, Gary (1989). *The Seat of the Soul*. New York. Simon and Schuster.

Index

20th Century social changes, 49, 81-83
21st Century elders
  connection, facilitating, 39
  mature expression of, 100-102, 182
  mobility of, 75
  as models, 190
  reengaging in life, 44
  roles of, 83-84, 90

accessibility, elders', 7-8, 56, 67, 80, 83
  and being verbal, 172-173
  and fear of mortality, 169
  giving attention, 181-183
  to grandchildren, 185-186
  and mobility, 19-20, 75, 129
  and retirement, 106, 144, 166
  and women, 31-32
adultism, 110-112
aged, bias against, 14-15, 62-63, 71-72, 186
aging, 36, 49-52 passim, 165-166
Albom, Mitch, 170
Ambrose, Saint, 112
American President [film], 96-97
ancestor worship, influence of, 53
ancient history, elders in, 45-66 passim
anima and animus, 100-101
archetypes, 15, 87, 91
  child/elder, male, 106-108
  childhood, 91, 104
  Crone, 48-49, 63, 88
  elder, 30, 87
  goddess, 48-49, 63
  Hero, 6-7, 86, 96, 133, 186, 189
  Lover, 87-90 passim, 93-95, 99, 103-104, 163, 175-176
  Magician, 57, 88, 90, 97-100, 163, 176
  Sovereign, 90, 91-93, 99-100, 163, 175-176
  Warrior, 89-91 passim, 95-97, 99-100, 133, 163, 176
  Wise Man, 67, 87, 88

Aristotle, 62-63
Arrien, Angeles, 148-149, 150
art as meditation, 113
ashramas, 25, 55
attention, giving, 182-183
Augustine, Saint, 66, 165-166
axis mundi, 92

balance, 102, 135, 175-177
  archetypal, 90
  fourfold, 1, 4, 17, 83-84, 130
  masculine and feminine energy, 67-68, 134, 176
  of needs and abilities, 56
  Puer and Senex, 106-107
  shadow and self-esteem, 133
Beach Music (Conroy), 147
Bible, 45-47, 51-52, 61, 93
bioenergetics, 40-41
births, out-of-wedlock, 100, 146, 173, 185, 195
Bismarck, Otto von, 35-36
blessing, original, 126
blessings by elders, 8-12, 24, 31, 126, 193-195
blessing way, 149, 182
Bly, Robert, 145-147, 150
Buber, Martin, 33-34, 81
Buddhism, 7-8, 33, 46, 63, 67, 68

Campbell, Joseph, 10, 13
career transition, 127
Carib customs, 57
celebrant role, 93, 163. *See also* blessings by elders
celebration, second half of life, 166-168
ceremonies, elder's role in. *See* blessings by elders
ceremony, elder incorporation, 161-164
chakras, 42
challenges, mid-life, 127-130
change, stages of, viii-ix, 152-153

child, elder as revived, 103-121
childhood environment, 108-110
children, elders and, 185-187
children, working, 129
China, 36, 40, 50, 53-55, 193-194. *See also* Taoism
Chinen, Allan, 30, 86
Christianity, 66-69 passim, 72-73, 123, 160. *See also* Bible
church elder, comparison with, 14
Cohen, Stanley, 40-41
community
    facilitation of, 183-185
    history-telling, 38
    individualism and, 55
    mobility and, 75
compassion, 59
competition, 25, 136-137
Confucianism, 53-54
Conroy, Pat, 147
conservationism. *See* earthkeeper role
container, holding the, 80
craftsmen, master, 18, 24-25, 31, 59
Creation Spirituality
    art as meditation, 113
    Four Paths, 5-7, 123-124
    original blessing, 126
    panentheism, 85
    social justice, 6, 82-83, 123
    work, reinvention of, 37
creativity, 119-121
credibility, aged's loss of, 18-27
Crone archetype, 48-49, 63, 88

Dark Ages, 26, 66, 68-69, 72, 112
Darwin, Charles, 24
dependence, mutual, 23
Desert Fathers and Mothers, 60, 62
discernment, 68, 80, 174-175
Donne, John, 72
dreams, honoring mentee's, 31, 32-33
DuBois, W.E.B, 195, 197

earthkeeper role, 5, 39-42, 56-57, 163, 190-191
Echhart, Meister, 5

education statistics, 132
ego
    compared with the soul, 28, 173
    egocentricity in elder, revived, 112
    and enlightenment, 7
    death of, 49
    integrity, 143, 144, 150
    loosening grip of, 173-175
elder
    archetype, 30, 87
    becoming an, 141-179
    compared with church elder, 14
    compared with elderly, 13-14, 21, 65-66, 189
    definition of, ix, 1-2, 17-18, 90
    role, 79-102
    within, 15, 49, 68-69, 171-172
Elder Council, 178-179
elderhood
    action in, 181-201
    growing into, 164-166
    sacredness of, 152-154
    as stage of personal growth, 142-151
elderly, ii, 104, 169, 189. *See also* elder: compared with elderly
Eliade, Mircea, 92
enclosure of people, 19, 44, 73, 130 138
energy, bright, 93, 95, 97, 99
energy, shadow. *See* shadow
enlightenment, 7, 55-56, 60, 113
Erikson, Eric, 20, 39
Erikson, Erik, 10, 105, 142-143, 146-147, 150
eros, 94
Estes, Clarissa Pinkola, 49
exercises
    elder-within meditation, 171-172
    initiation questions, 156
    listing your roles, 173
    Severe Teachers banquet, 168-169

facilitator of journey, elder as, 7-8
family
    advocating for, 185-187

Index

family, *continued*
  industrialization and, 23, 25, 35
  story-telling, 38, 39
  See also filial piety
Far Eastern elderhood, 53-56
Farrell, Warren, 82, 137
fasting, 157, 159
fatherhood. *See* parenting: men and
fatherlessness, 132, 146, 185, 195
feminine energy, 67-68, 100-102, 190
femininity, mature, 127
feminist consciousness, 131, 134
filial piety, 53-54
First Knight [film], 92-93
Fisher King [film], 94
forgiveness, importance of, 168-169
Four Paths, 5-7, 123-124
fourfold balance, viii, 1, 4, 83-84, 130, 165
Fox, Matthew, iv, 4, 5, 85, 123
Freud, Sigmund, 20, 64, 94

Gaia, 41, 42
Gandhi, Mahatma, 4, 91
gender
  differences, viii, 132, 137
  roles, 25, 81-84, 90, 129, 138-140
generativity, 2, 3, 6, 143, 186
  Erikson on, 143, 150
  and family, 187
  and mentoring, 34
  restraints on, 69, 77, 130
  and retirement, 143-144
  Sovereign energy and, 175
  and time, 106
  and *thanatos*, 181
gerontocracy, 19, 70, 76
gerontophobia, 76
Gibran, Kahlil, 12, 20, 95
Gillette, Douglas, 149-151
goddess archetype, 48-49, 63
Goethe, Johann, 170
Goldberg, Herb, 136
good work, 18, 37, 72
Greek mythology, 63
grounded, being, 40-41
Gurdjieff, G.I, 51

harvesting, 37, 70, 133, 166, 191-192, 193
health, modeling, 188-189
Heard, Gerald, 29
Hebrew scriptures, 14, 45, 51-52, 67
Heidi (Spyri), 114-119
hermits, 60-61
Hero archetype, 6-7, 86, 96, 133, 186, 189
Herodotus, 50
Hesse, Hermann, 33
Hildegard of Bingen, 66, 98
Hillman, James, 6
Hinduism, 25, 42, 54-55, 60, 63, 119
holding the container, 80-81, 105, 178, 196
Homer, 63
Hun, 53
husbandry, 19, 130

immaturity, 128, 132-133, 134-140, 146
immigration, effects of, 19-20, 76
impoverishment, spiritual, 43-44, 91, 130, 132-133, 144-145
incorporation phase, 155, 161-164
India, 25, 54-55, 61
indigenous societies' customs, 56-60
Industrial Era, 23-27
  decline of mentoring, 30
  enclosure, 73
  feminist consciousness, 131
  immaturity, 128-130
  public education, 65
  and social security, 36
  as shock stage, viii
  women's roles, 19, 25, 138
  work for income, 26
  See also immigration, effects of;
    machines, effects of using
initiation of an elder, 151-164
initiations, 10-12, 24, 98, 200. *See also* blessings by elders
inner elder. *See* elder: within
Iron John (Bly), 145-147

Joseph, Jenny, 120
Judaism, 46, 52, 63

215

Jung, Carl, 73, 80, 84-86, 90, 106-107

Kenobi, Ben (Obi-Wan), 98
Kimura, Doreen, 137
Kipling, Rudyard, 168
Knudtsen, Peter, 56-57
Krause, Karl, 85

labor statistics, 129, 132
lama, 46, 61
leadership, passing on, 187-188
legacy, passing on, 198-199
libido, 20-21, 64, 81, 94, 156, 165-166, 198
life completion planning, 127
life history, recording one's, 38-39
life review, 167-168
life span, 45, 52, 66, 72
lila, 119
longevity, 3, 36, 45, 52
Lover energy. *See* archetypes, Lover
Luther, Martin, 72

machines, effects of using, 135-136
magic and elderhood, 49-50
Magician energy. *See* archetypes: Magician
mantle of elderhood, 128, 155, 162-165 passim
Marcel, Gabriel, 69, 75
masculine energy, 67-68, 100-102, 190
masculine mystique, 131, 134-135, 137, 139, 189. *See also* competition
masculinity, re-definition of, 81-82, 139
maturity, 90-91, 112, 123-140, 147
Mead, Margaret, 125-126, 188
Mechtild of Magdeburg, 69
meditation, elder-within, 171-172
Meetings With Remarkable Men (Gurdjieff), 51
menopause and wisdom, 48
men's gatherings, vii, 10
mentoring, iv, ix, 2, 30-35, 198-200
    and accessibility, 182
    and balance, 124
    history, 25, 61, 76, 129

hunger for, 18
and knowledge of the whole, 58
Magician archetype and, 103
Robert Bly on, 145-147 passim
Minois, George, 112
mobility and immobility, 75, 129
Moore, Robert, 149-151
moral development, 34-35, 44, 46, 60, 85, 142
mortality, 20, 64, 71, 127, 144, 150, 169-171
Moses, 14, 45-47, 53, 55, 60
motherhood. *See* parenting: women and
Myth of Male Power (Farrell), 82
mythology, 63, 86
Native American customs, 59
Newest Age, 29, 37, 43-44, 111, 118
nirvana, 7

oral tradition, 50-53, 56, 59
Origen, 112

pace, setting a nourishing, 191-193
panentheism, 85
parenting
    men and, 62, 65, 132, 139-140, 146, 185-186
    responsibilities, 55
    women and, 27, 35, 47, 146
parents as elders. *See* blessings by elders
patriarchy (*pater familias*)
    decline of, 61-62, 134, 176
    father's rights in, 63-66
    father's role in, 34-35
    feminist movement and, 131
    rise of, 47
peai, 57
Peter Pan and Captain Hook, 107
Piaget, Jean, 10
play, 119-121
Plutarch, 64
power, 131-132, 134-135, 176
pre-Industrial Era communities, 23, 74

prejudices, seeing beyond, 195-196
present, focus in the, 48
prestige and aging, 49-50, 51, 52
property ownership and status, 22
Prophet, The (Gibran), 12, 20
protector role, 47, 83-84, 93, 99, 139, 189-191
provider role, 84, 99-100, 139, 182-185, 188-189
psyche, 15, 33, 85-87, 90, 123, 130, 133
  and archetypes, 91, 98, 102, 103
  Bly on, 146-147
  See also anima and animus; elder within; energy, bright; feminine energy; masculine energy; shadow; protector role; provider role; teacher role; yin and yang
psychic energies, balancing, 175-177
Puer, 106-107

rebbe, 46
recreation as re-creating, 166-167
Red Hat Society, 120-121
reframing, 167-168, 169
religion, 4, 62, 86, 153
Renaissance elders, 70-73
respect for elders, decline of, 61-64
retirement, 35-37, 44, 72, 76, 106, 143-145, 197-199
retreat, going on, 159
Return of the King (Tolkein), 88
Rich, Adrienne, 131
rites of passage. *See* initiations; blessings by elders
ritual elder, 98, 158, 161-162
roles, 79-102
  as archetypes, 84-87
  celebrant, 93, 163 (*see also* blessings by elders)
  earthkeeper, 5, 39-42, 56-57, 163, 190-191
  exercise listing, 173
  gender, 25, 81-84, 90, 129, 138-140
  mentor, 30-35, 129, 163, 182, 199, 200
  wisdomkeeper, 37-39, 163, 201

roles, *continued*
  See also protector role; provider role; teacher role
Romans, 47, 49, 52-53, 64, 65, 66, 93
roshi, 46
Rousseau, Jean-Jacques, 140
Rumi, 6, 127-128

sacred space, 9-10, 158-159, 182, 184-185, 192, 195-196
sacredness, 164
sage, 1, 46, 69, 80, 59, 198-199
Sanhedrin, 61
sannyassin, 55, 56, 61
Schachter-Shalomi, Rabbi Zalman, 13, 166
self to other, movement of, 35, 151
Senex, 106-107
separation phase, 154, 156-157
Service Corps of Retired Executives (SCORE), 200
service, elderhood as, 63-66, 72, 127
shadow, 90, 93-99 passim, 133, 168, 175-177
Shakespeare, William, 71, 104
shamanism, 57-58, 99
sheikh, 46
Siddhartha, Guatama, 33
Simmons, Leo, 197
simplification of life, 56, 60-61
Smith, Adam, 24
social justice, 6, 82-83, 126
Social Security system, 36
Socrates, 55-56, 80, 98
Sophia, 67
soul, 4-5, 128
  elder expression of, 7, 15, 16, 31
  historical effects on, 73, 75, 76-77, 128, 130
  nourishment, 81, 135, 183, 191-193
  and work, viii, 27-29, 135-136
  See also eros; Hun
Sovereign energy. *See* archetypes, Sovereign
spirit, 3-6, 66, 74, 77, 85-86, 113, 117

Spiritual Eldering Institute, iii, 168-169, 171-172
spiritual elders, xi, 1-42, 170
spiritual journey, xi, 1, 3-8, 16-17, 37, 191. *See also* ego: loosening grip of; self to other, movement of
Spyri, Joanna, 114
stages of personal development, 42, 69, 125, 126, 142-151, 170. *See also* ashramas; initiations
Star Wars [film], 98-99
staretz, 46, 61
stewardship, ix, 1, 99, 149, 150, 190-191
Sufism, 8, 68
supernatural powers, 49-50, 98
Suzuki, David, 56-57, 58-59

Taoism, 54, 68, 87
teacher role, 81, 84, 100, 198
   Magician archetype and, 97, 100
   and mandatory education, 65
   Severe Teachers, 168-169
   in various cultures, 7-8, 55
   See also mentoring; wisdomkeeper role
thanatos, 20-21, 64, 81, 156, 195, 198
Thoreau, Henry David, 14-15, 39, 74, 106
threshold phase, 154, 157-161
Thurman, Howard, 3
Tolkein, J.R.R, 88-89
transition phases, 152, 153
tsu, 53, 54
Tuesdays With Morrie (Albom), 170
Turner, Frederick, 21-22

unconscious, 49, 80-81, 85-86, 100, 119, 168. *See also* archetypes: Magician; shadow
University of Creation Spirituality, iv, 113
useless elder, 181-182

van Gennep, Arnold, 11, 164
Via Creativa, Via Negativa, Via Positiva, Via Transformativa. *See* Four Paths
victims of progress, elders as, 27-29
village commons, 23, 26, 31, 73, 129
vision quest, 161
volunteering, 196-197, 200

wage statistics, 132
Warrior energy. *See* archetypes: Warrior
Wells, H.G, 72
wisdom, 166, 169
   age versus, 52-53, 58
   developing confidence in, 171-173
   historical views of, 67-69
   and menopause, 48
   tools of, 158-159, 168
wisdomkeeper role, 37-39, 67, 163, 201
Wisdom of the Elders (Suzuki and Knudtson), 56-58
Wise Man archetype, 67, 87, 88
Wollstonecraft, Mary, 131
women's gatherings, 10-11, 49
work, reinvention of, 37
World War II, 76-77
working for income, 26

Yeats, William, 124
yin and *yang*, 68, 87
youth, elders challenged by, 62-64

About the Author

2006 is the 35 year anniversary of marriage of the author to his wife Linda and was also the year of birth of Terry's seventh grandchild. Among his top priorities in this, his 66th year are grandparenting, leading eldering workshops, maintaining an involvement in men's work, doing spiritual direction and writing.

Terry has graduate degrees in history and counseling and received his Doctorate in Ministry in 2005. He founded the Elderhood Institute in 2001 when he retired from management of EASE the mental health consulting firm he formed in 1979.

Terry's first book was co-authored with Paul Kadota: *A Biography of Kanaye Nagasawa*. It is about a Japanese-American adventurer, entrepreneur and spiritual leader and was published in Kagoshima, Japan in 1978. He is also the author of *Also of Men Born*, EASE Inc. 1996 and *Employee Assistance Programs in Industry*, a pamphlet published by the Do It Now Foundation, Phoenix, 1980.

In 2001 Bookpartners of Oregon published Terry's first book on elderhood, *The Elder Within*.